Advance Praise for the *Flavor without FODMAPs Cookbook*

"The wonderful menus in the *Flavor without FODMAPs Cookbook* enticed me into the kitchen. After a week of cooking and baking, I am proud to say these recipes are delicious, easy, and everyone in the family loves them! I love not having to apologize for low-FODMAP foods. I can entertain with these recipes and no one will be the wiser. I'm not a natural cook, so I appreciate the detailed advice about how to modify recipes for a low-FODMAP diet. And of course the updated low-FODMAP food lists are invaluable." – *Lauren Pulver*

"While this book does acknowledge high-FODMAP foods to eliminate, the focus is on delicious, nutritious foods that patients on a low-FODMAP diet *can* eat, with emphasis on variety and expanding the diet as much as possible. This approach is key for achieving long term success and satisfaction. Sample menus are balanced and complete. Most recipes are easy to follow, quick to prepare, and use common ingredients. I would strongly recommend this book to IBS patients who have been prescribed a low-FODMAP diet to help them spend less time figuring out what to eat and more time enjoying their food." – *Shirley Paski, MD, Gastroenterologist*

"As an experienced and adventurous cook, I haven't had a lot of trouble adapting my own recipes to the low-FODMAP lifestyle. However, there is something to be said for owning a cookbook that is completely geared to my dietary needs, with recipes I don't have to think about. This is the beauty of Patsy Catsos' new cookbook. Not only are her recipes all elimination-friendly, they are also food-lover friendly and nutritionally balanced. There are a variety of options for vegetarians, from vegetables and eggs to healthy grains, tempeh and tofu. The baked goods are especially exciting to me, as most of the gluten-free flour blends on the market are full of gums and other ingredients I don't choose to consume. Patsy's baked goods are real food with actual nutritional value. This cookbook appeals to me first as a foodie (as it should), and second as a low-FODMAP addition to my library. I'm looking forward to cooking my way through it." – *Lisa Braithwaite, Public Speaking Coach and Trainer*

"In the *Flavor without FODMAPs Cookbook* Patsy has taken the guesswork out of following a low-FODMAP diet by providing all the tools you will need. From setting up a pantry, to label reading tips, menus, special occasion meals and an incredible number of delicious recipes, this book has it all." – Marlisa Brown, MS, RD, CDE, CDN, author of *Gluten-Free, Hassle-Free* and *Easy, Gluten-Free*

"As the mom of two kids with digestive disorders, including fructose malabsorption and IBS, I've relied on Patsy for her FODMAP expertise since she wrote her first book, *IBS—Free at Last*! When she told me she had a cookbook in the works I almost couldn't contain my excitement. I cannot wait to share this cookbook with my fructose malabsorption support group and with family and friends who struggle with IBS." – *Erin Cox, Administrator, Parents of FructMal Kids USA Facebook Group*

Flavor without FODMAPs Cookbook

Love the Foods that Love You Back

Patsy Catsos, M.S., R.D.N., L.D.

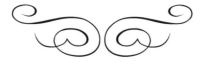

This publication contains the opinions and ideas of its author. It is intended to provide helpful information on how certain individuals can minimize IBS symptoms by manipulating their intake of dietary carbohydrates. It is sold with the understanding that the author is not engaged in rendering medical, health, or any other kind of personal or professional services. Readers are urged to share the information in this book with a health care provider before adopting any of the suggestions. Readers are advised to discuss symptoms with a medical adviser and not use this book to self-diagnose IBS. The author and publisher specifically disclaim all responsibility for any liability, loss, or risk, personal or otherwise, incurred as a consequence, directly or indirectly, from the use or application of any of the contents of this book.

Pond Cove Press, P.O. Box 10106, Portland, ME 04104-0106

ISBN: 0-9820635-3-9

ISBN-13: 978-0-9820635-3-8

Order additional copies at www.CreateSpace.com
Cover image © Patsy Catsos
Cover design by Shirley Douglas

Table of Contents

INTRODUCTION

"I love onions, but they don't love me back." If this sounds like the story of your life, you may be sensitive to the FODMAPs in food, as many folks with irritable bowel syndrome (IBS) are. In fact, up to 75% of people with IBS get relief from their IBS symptoms on a low FODMAP diet. You can learn more about IBS and FODMAPs in the next chapter, but for the moment, let's just say that many people with symptoms of gas, bloating, abdominal pain, diarrhea, and/or constipation feel a whole lot better if they eat less of foods such as

- Milk and yogurt
- Apples, pears, peaches, blackberries, watermelon, fruit juice, and dried fruit of all kinds
- Wheat and rye in all forms, including bread, pasta, crackers, bagels, pizza, muffins, and breakfast cereal
- Onions, garlic, corn, cauliflower, and mushrooms
- Beans, hummus, and soy milk
- High-fiber bars, cereals and breads
- Smoothies and shakes
- Nuts and trail mix

"Wait," you protest. "I eat those foods because they are healthy. I deliberately eat lots of them. And they are in *everything I cook!*" When I hear these protests from one of my IBS patients, I think, "Yes, and that might explain a few things." These very foods can cause bouts of IBS symptoms to occur. I agree, they are good for you, but only up to the point where they cause you pain and distress. You can conduct a dietary experiment to learn how FODMAPs affect you by eating only low-FODMAP foods for a few weeks, then reintroducing high-FODMAP foods and monitoring your symptoms. If you need help planning your FODMAP elimination and challenge, seek help from a registered dietitian nutritionist (R.D. or R.D.N.) with expertise in the FODMAP approach or check my web site, www.ibsfree.net, for more resources.

Some of you may nod your heads knowingly as you read the above list of foods. You've been aware some of these foods cause gastrointestinal distress, and you avoid them. Maybe you've put yourself on a dairy-free or gluten-free diet and noticed you feel better. It will be interesting for you to learn more about FODMAPs because it will explain and confirm your own observations. The FODMAP approach may help you liberalize your diet if you find you can tolerate low-lactose dairy products, or that gluten isn't the culprit in wheat that you thought it was. Discovering other foods you are likely to tolerate will add variety and interest to your meals and make it much easier to dine at restaurants or dinner parties.

I wrote this cookbook to make your low-FODMAP journey a pleasant one. It can be difficult to relearn to cook without your go-to kitchen staples, and not everyone lives next door to a grocery store with a full line of specialty foods. I hope it will make your life easier to have a cookbook designed with your needs in mind, in which each and every recipe is suitable for a low-FODMAP diet. This book celebrates flavor without FODMAPs and will help you:

- Easily make home-made alternatives for hard-to-find commercially prepared foods.
- Learn how your favorite recipes can be adapted to be more gut-friendly.
- Prepare food that tastes so good, no one will need to know you are on a special diet.
- Have more fun when you are planning special occasions.

In the years since I published the first edition of my book, *IBS—Free at Last!*, I have interacted with thousands of patients and readers. One thing is increasingly apparent: citizens of the world today are passionate about their food. People identify very strongly with their food philosophies. In the past, with limited interaction and travel outside the local community, people had little choice but to eat like their neighbors. With exotic food and health information streaming to and from almost every corner of the world, food trends and philosophies are emerging quickly. I want to make sure you understand my point of view so you can decide whether this is the right cookbook for you. I don't believe there is one perfect diet for good health. I believe that humans are biologically omnivores and that anything edible is fair game as food, at least for healthy people. In this day and age, many of us choose to limit our intake of certain food groups for social, political, or religious reasons, but as a dietitian and a cook, I don't abhor eating meat or dairy or gluten or anything else just on principle. My job as a dietitian is to encourage each person within his or her own value system to eat the widest variety of nutritious, well-tolerated foods. The spirit of the FODMAP elimination and challenge process is experimental, not rule-bound. All this is to say that the recipes in this cookbook are all low in FODMAPs, and they are made from a wide variety of whole, real foods. The rest of your food philosophy is up to you.

- **If you are on a FODMAP elimination diet**, you will be pleased to learn that every single recipe in this book is suitable for the elimination phase of the diet, according to information available as of the date of publication. Hurray! No modifications are necessary to make them suitable for a low-FODMAP diet in the portions shown, for otherwise healthy omnivores.
- **If you've been through the process of FODMAP challenges with your dietitian (or with my book, *IBS—Free at Last!*)and have identified some types of FODMAPs that don't bother you,** you can modify these recipes back toward more conventional ingredients and preparation. For example, if you learn that you are not lactose

intolerant, then by all means use regular fluid milk in any of these recipes instead of lactose-free milk. Or if you've found that you can tolerate onions without a problem, feel free to add them or to substitute them for an equal quantity of other vegetables called for in one of these recipes.

- **If you find you must limit or avoid certain FODMAPs over a longer period of time,** this book can anchor your collection of new recipes.

- **If you are a vegan, don't buy this cookbook** unless you are prepared to make some additional modifications on your own. Because lactose-free milk products and cheeses are low in FODMAPs, great sources of protein and calcium, and enjoyed by many people, recipes in this book often call for butter, cheese, and milk. I have, however, included a few vegan recipes.

- **People with IBS run the gamut in terms of their caloric needs,** and the recipes in this book vary accordingly. Some of the special occasion recipes in this book are quite rich, and unless you need to gain weight (which some people with IBS do), you should probably use them sparingly. When milk is called for in the recipes, please choose the type of lactose-free milk (non-fat, low-fat, whole) that is appropriate for your caloric needs. Nutrients were calculated using low-fat cow's milk unless otherwise specified.

- **If you have other medical conditions, take certain medications, or have food allergies,** you may have to further modify these recipes. For example, if you have inflammatory bowel disease or gastroparesis, you may have to adjust the fiber or fat content of the diet. If you take blood thinners, you may have to modify your intake of leafy greens. If you need help with modifications, please consult a registered dietitian nutritionist. Never eat a food to which you are allergic, even if it appears in one of the menus or recipes in this book.

FODMAP ELIMINATION DIET: NUTSHELL VERSION

This short chapter will briefly lay out the basics of the low-FODMAP elimination diet and challenge process. A FODMAP elimination diet is a learning diet. It is not meant to be a permanent way of eating. You start by eating only low-FODMAP foods, such as the ones in your low-FODMAP pantry. A low-FODMAP diet helps about 75 percent of people with IBS get satisfactory relief of their symptoms. If the diet is going to help you, you should start to feel better within a few weeks. Next, you carefully add FODMAPs back to your diet. By paying close attention to your symptoms, you will learn which FODMAPs are triggers for your IBS (so that you can limit or avoid them), as well as which you are able to tolerate.

If the term "FODMAP" is new to you, you are not alone. FODMAP is the acronym for **F**ermentable **O**ligo-, **D**i-, and **M**ono-saccharides **A**nd **P**olyols. Don't let this awkward term scare you away. You don't have to be a biochemist to eat a low-FODMAP diet. I've studied the science so you don't have to. Here are the important parts:

FODMAP carbohydrates include certain natural *sugars* in foods such as milk, fruit, honey, and high-fructose corn syrup. FODMAPs also include certain *fibers* in foods such as wheat, onions, garlic, and beans. (Speaking of wheat, note that gluten is not a FODMAP—it's just a coincidence than FODMAPs and gluten coexist in wheat, as well as in rye and barley.) The load of FODMAPs from all sources have a cumulative effect. Examples of FODMAPs include:

- Lactose (also known as milk sugar, found in milk, yogurt, and ice cream)
- Fructose (also known as fruit sugar, found in fruit, high-fructose corn syrup, honey, and agave syrup)
- Sugar alcohols such as sorbitol, mannitol, and other "-ol" sweeteners (found in certain fruits and vegetables, as well as some types of sugar-free gums and candies); sugar alcohols are sometimes known as polyols
- Oligosaccharides (sometimes referred to as fructans and GOS, these are fibers found in wheat, onions, garlic, chicory root, beans, hummus, and soy milk)

All FODMAP carbohydrates have a few things in common:

- They may be poorly absorbed in the small intestine. Instead, as the hours go by after a meal, these sugars and fibers linger in the small intestine, then move along into the large intestine.
- They are the favorite foods of the normal bacteria that live in the intestines. When these bacteria eat FODMAPs, the process of fermentation creates a lot of gas.
- FODMAPs can act like a sponge to pull extra water into the gut and disrupt fluid

balance.

With a little imagination, you can picture the combination of gas and fluid causing the intestines to swell up like a water balloon. People with IBS experience this as a painful bloating sensation. They may pass an excessive amount of gas or have urgent watery diarrhea, constipation, or both.

Bacterial fermentation is actually a normal part of life and produces some substances that are valuable to our health. The intention of the FODMAP elimination and challenge process is not to stamp out fermentation altogether, but to keep it at a manageable level. Keep in mind your eventual goal is to eat the most varied and nutritious diet *you* can tolerate. I encourage you to do the best you can to reintroduce valuable high-FODMAP foods when you are ready.

The FODMAP concept was originated by researchers at Box Hill Hospital and Monash University in Australia, including Susan J. Shepherd, Peter R. Gibson, Jacqueline S. Barrett, and Jane Muir. This group continues to publish most of the emerging FODMAP food composition data. If you live in their part of the world, you might be interested in the excellent low-FODMAP diet material, shopping guides, and cookbooks published by the Eastern Health Clinical School at Monash University and by ShepherdWorks. Sales of the Monash University smartphone apps help fund ongoing FODMAP research.

The food lists and teaching tools I've developed are based on the available data about the FODMAP content of foods at the time of publication. However, you can expect some minor variations from one teaching tool and set of recipes to the next. Each tool and project team filters the FODMAP data through a different lens, and that's okay. A few minor discrepancies don't diminish the impact of lowering the overall FODMAP load of your diet. For example, I tend to decide if a food is low enough in FODMAPs based upon the amount of FODMAPs in a standard serving size, such as ½ cup of vegetables, while another system might shrink the portion down to a very small size if necessary to give the food a "green light."

Detailed guidance on the elimination and re-challenge process is outside the scope of this book. Seek help from a knowledgeable registered dietitian nutritionist or see www.ibsfree.net for links to other publications that can assist you.

YOUR LOW-FODMAP PANTRY

To pull off a successful FODMAP elimination diet, you've got to have low-FODMAP foods on hand when it's time to make your next meal. Stock your pantry and refrigerator with some of these staples and you'll be prepared. In all cases, buy a brand that does not contain FODMAP ingredients. For example, jam is in the pantry, but it must be jam made from low-FODMAP fruit such as blueberries and sweetened with a low-FODMAP sweetener like sugar. Because manufacturers change ingredients frequently, please read the label *every time* to check for FODMAPs. Ingredients and brand names change frequently, so I have not listed brand names in the pantry. Instead, I've done two things:

- I've placed an asterisk (*) after the items that often contain questionable ingredients and are your highest label-reading priorities. These are all processed foods. The easiest way to make sure your foods don't contain FODMAPs is to choose the fresh whole foods listed instead of food that comes in bottles, cans, or boxes.
- I have developed a Pinterest board with low-FODMAP, brand name grocery items. You don't have to have a Pinterest account yourself to visit me at www.pinterest.com/pcatsos. When you view my Pinterest boards, you can see pictures of brand name groceries that are suitable for a low-FODMAP diet.

Some of the foods in the pantry will be new to you. You don't have to eat them if you don't want to, especially if you are doing a short-term elimination diet. However, if you find yourself following a low-FODMAP diet over a more extended time period, these alternative foods can expand your culinary horizons. A more varied diet offers a wider variety of nutrients, too.

Some of the items in your low-FODMAP pantry do have small amounts of FODMAPs in them. For best results, you should only eat one or two portions of those foods at a time; **look for the bold font and note the recommended portion.** Other (non-bold) foods can be consumed according to your caloric needs and appetite. As researchers learn more about the FODMAP content of foods, FODMAP status and/or portions may change. If you have read *IBS—Free at Last!* with publication dates of 2009 or 2012, the lists of low-FODMAP foods in this chapter supersede those published previously.

Be sure to modify these food lists to suit your other health conditions. For example, people with gluten-related disorders should not eat foods containing gluten, such as sourdough-spelt bread, and should use only gluten-free versions of foods on this list such as oats, breakfast cereals, tempeh, and soy sauce. There are many other conditions, too numerous to list, that require dietary modification. Please seek help from a registered dietitian to modify these food lists as needed.

Grains and Starches

Amaranth

Breakfast cereals, cold, made of rice or corn, ½ cup*

Breakfast cereals, cold, made of buckwheat, quinoa, amaranth or millet*

Buckwheat cereal, hot

Buckwheat flour

Soba noodles*

Oatmeal, ¼ cup dry or ½ cup cooked*

Oat bran, dry, 1 tablespoon

Oat flour, ¼ cup

Gluten-free pretzels*

Gluten-free bread*

Grits

Corn, rice or quinoa pasta*

Corn tortillas, 6-inch*

Corn or tortilla chips*

Crackers, rice or corn*

Cornmeal

Millet

Polenta

Popcorn

Potatoes, white

Potato chips*

Quinoa

Rice or popcorn cakes*

Rice, brown or white

Rice bran

Rice cereal, hot

Sorghum

Sourdough-spelt bread*

Wild rice

Tip: Avoid seasoned grain mixes. Gluten, the protein

Fruits

Banana, ½

Blueberries, ½ cup

Blueberry juice, ½ cup

Cantaloupe, ½ cup

Clementine, 1 medium

Coconut, shredded, ½ cup

Cranberries, raw, ½ cup

Cranberry juice, ½ cup*

Dragon fruit, ½ cup

Durian, ½ cup

Grapes, all kinds, ½ cup

Grape juice, ½ cup

Honeydew, ½ cup

Kiwi, 1 medium

Orange juice, ½ cup

Orange, 1 small

Papaya, ½ cup

Pineapple, ½ cup

Prickly pear fruit, 1

Raspberries, ½ cup

Rhubarb, ½ cup

Strawberries, ½ cup

Tangelo, 1 medium

Tips: Limit fruit to 1 serving per meal or snack. Choose fresh or frozen fruit. No dried fruit, fruit juice drinks or fruit juice other than those listed.

LEGEND:

*	Read the label and avoid processed foods that have FODMAP ingredients added.
Bold	Contains a small amount of FODMAPs. For best results, do not exceed the portion size shown.

Vegetables

Alfalfa sprouts
Arugula/rocket
Bamboo shoots
Bean sprouts
Bok choy, ½ cup
Butternut squash, ½ cup
Cabbage, common, ½ cup
Carrots
Cherry tomatoes
Chicory leaves
Chili pepper, red
Cucumber
Eggplant
Endive
Fennel bulb, ½ cup
Green beans, ½ cup
Green bell peppers
Green peas, ½ cup
Kabocha squash
Kale, 1 cup raw or ½ cup cooked
Leek, leaves only

Leaf lettuce
Okra, ½ cup
Parsnip
Pattypan squash
Pickle, dill or sour
Radishes
Red bell pepper
Scallions/green onions, green part only
Seaweed/nori
Spinach
Summer squash
Sweet potato, ½ cup
Tomato, canned, whole or diced
Tomato, fresh
Turnip/rutabaga, ½ cup
Water chestnuts
Zucchini

Tip: Choose fresh vegetables or frozen vegetables without sauce.

Nuts and Seeds

Almonds, 2 tablespoons
Almond butter, 2 tablespoons
Chia seeds, 2 tablespoons
Macadamia nuts, 2 tablespoons
Peanuts, 2 tablespoons
Peanut butter, 2 tablespoons
Pecans, 2 tablespoons
Pine nuts, 2 tablespoons

Pumpkin seeds/pepitas, 2 tablespoons
Sesame seeds, 2 tablespoons
Sunflower seeds, 2 tablespoons
Walnuts, 2 tablespoons

Tip: Choose raw nuts/seeds or roasted, unseasoned nuts/seeds. Two tablespoon equals one small handful.

Oils

Coconut cream, canned, ½ cup
Coconut milk, canned, ¾ cup
Margarine
Mayonnaise*

Oil, any type, including olive , soybean, coconut, and garlic-infused
Tartar sauce*

Milk Fats

Butter
Cream cheese, 2 tablespoons*
Half-and-half, 2 tablespoons

Heavy cream, whipped, ¼ cup*
Sour cream, 2 tablespoons*

Meat/Fish/Poultry/Eggs

Beef
Buffalo
Chicken
Duck
Egg whites
Egg, whole
Fish, any kind
Goat

Lamb
Pork
Seafood, any kind
Turkey

Tip: Choose unseasoned, unbreaded, minimally-processed or ground meat, fish, and poultry

Plant-Based Proteins

Chickpeas/garbanzos, canned, drained, ½ cup
Lentils, canned, drained, rinsed, ½ cup
Lentils, red or green, cooked, drained, ½ cup
Quorn (Grounds only)*
Tempeh*

Tofu*

Tip: Choose medium or firm tofu that has been pressed and drained; silken tofu is not suitable.

Cow's Milk and Milk Products

Cheese, American, 1 ounce
Cheese, hard, regular or reduced-fat including Cheddar, Swiss, Parmesan, Brie, mozzarella, feta
Cottage cheese, lactose-free*
Dry curd cottage cheese

Goat cheese/chevre, 1 ounce
Kefir, lactose-free*
Milk, lactose-free
Ricotta cheese, regular, ⅓ cup
Yogurt, lactose-free*

Beverages

Beer
Black tea, weak, 8 fluid ounces
Chai tea, weak, 8 fluid ounces*
Coconut water
Coffee, black, filtered
Dandelion tea, weak, 8 fluid ounces*
Espresso, black
Green tea

Peppermint tea
Spirits (not rum)
Rice milk*
White tea, 8 fluid ounces
Wine, red or white (not sherry or port)

Tip: Alcohol and caffeine can affect gut function even in low-FODMAP beverages; consume in moderation.

Sweets

Brown rice syrup, 1 ½ tablespoons
Candy/chocolate made with allowed ingredients, 1 ounce*
Cane syrup, 1 ½ tablespoons
Chocolate, semi-sweet, 1 ounce*
Corn syrup (not high-fructose), 1 ½ tablespoons
Golden syrup, 1 ½ tablespoons

Ice cream, lactose-free, ½ cup*
Jam or jelly, 1 ½ tablespoons*
Maple syrup, 100% pure (not "pancake" syrup), 1 ½ tablespoons
Sorbet, ½ cup*
Sugar: brown, cane, palm, confectioner's, granulated, 1 ½ tablespoons

Condiments and Seasonings

Allspice
Basil
Bay leaf
Black pepper
Chives, green part only
Cilantro
Cocoa powder, 1 ½ tablespoons
Coriander
Dill
Dry mustard powder
Fish sauce
Five spice
Garlic scapes
Garlic-infused oil (no garlic

"extract")
Ginger
Ground chile powder (100% chiles, not a blend)
Cumin
Italian seasoning*
Lemon or lime juice
Marjoram
Mustard, prepared
Olives
Oregano
Paprika
Parsley
Poultry seasoning*

Rosemary
Salt
Scallions (green part only)
Sesame oil, toasted or spicy
Soy sauce
Tamari*
Turmeric
Vinegar, balsamic, 2 tablespoons
Vinegar, other types

Tip: Choose single ingredient fresh or dried herbs.

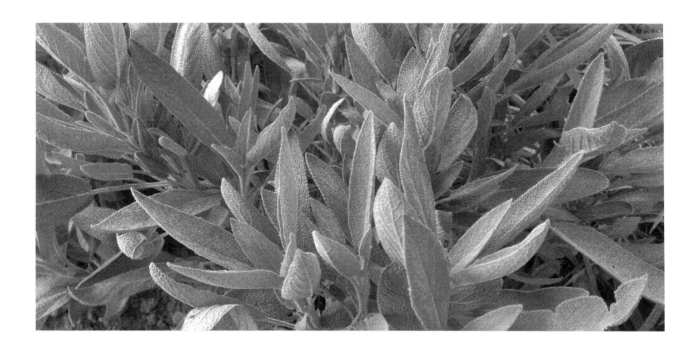

LABEL READING TIPS

The ingredients below are considered low in FODMAPs at the time of this writing. That is not to say they are all "healthy choices," and I am not endorsing their use by listing them here. What's right for one person may not be right for another. For example, while I don't endorse the use of aspartame, I am sharing the information about its FODMAP status with you so you can make an informed decision about whether or not you want to consume it. Likewise, gluten or sucralose may have effects on GI function, but they are not FODMAPs. Gums are another group of additives that do not meet the definition of FODMAPs, but may, nonetheless, be poorly tolerated. Of course, you may choose to omit any of these ingredients or additives if you wish. With the exception of salt, none is an essential part of the diet. If in doubt, please discuss appropriate choices with your dietitian.

Aspartame
Baker's yeast
Baking powder
Baking soda
Bar sugar
Barley malt
Beet sugar
Berry sugar
Black pepper
Brown sugar
Brown rice syrup
Cane juice crystals
Cane sugar
Cane syrup
Carageenan
Castor sugar
Cocoa butter
Confectioner's sugar
Cornstarch
Corn syrup (not high-fructose)
Corn syrup solids

Cultured corn syrup
Dehydrated sugar cane juice
Demerara sugar
Dextrose
Gellan gum
Glucose
Gluten
Granulated sugar
Guar gum
Gum Acacia
Gum Arabic
High-maltose corn syrup
Icing sugar
Invert sugar
Malt extract
Maltodextrin
Maltose
Modified food starch
Organic sugar
Palm sugar
Pectin

Raw sugar
Refined sugar
Resistant starch
Saccharine
Salt
Soy lecithin
Soybean oil
Spelt flour
Stevia
Sucrose
Sugar
Sugar syrup
Superfine sugar
Sucralose
Tapioca
Tara gum
Vital wheat gluten
Wheat starch
Whey protein isolate
Xanthan gum

I do NOT recommend these foods and ingredients on a low-FODMAP diet. Please keep in mind that a FODMAP elimination diet is meant to be a short-term learning diet, not a permanent way of eating. While some of these foods are no great loss nutritionally speaking, many of them contain valuable nutrients. After a few weeks on a low-FODMAP diet, make an effort to reintroduce these fruits, vegetables, beans and whole grains as tolerated. The best way to do this is to follow a reintroduction schedule designed to help you figure out your level of tolerance to each type of FODMAP. Details on that process are outside the scope of this book. Please visit my website, www.ibsfree.net, for resources, including a directory of registered dietitians familiar with the FODMAP elimination and challenge process and links to my book, *IBS—Free at Last!*

Please note that this is not a complete list of foods that contain FODMAPs, because our knowledge base is still incomplete. There can be discrepancies between the specific foods listed on various teaching tools. These can occur when tools become outdated or because the creators of the tools make different choices about portions sizes or cut-offs for what is considered high-FODMAP. Cut-off levels for FODMAPs are based on clinical experience and have not yet been validated in clinical trials. Sugar-free foods containing sorbitol, maltitol, xylitol , erythritol and other sugar alcohols are not suitable for a low-FODMAP diet. They are referred to as "-ol sweeteners" on this list.

Agave nectar
Agave syrup
All-purpose flour
Apple cider
Apple juice
Apple sauce
Apples, fresh or dried
Apricot nectar
Apricots, fresh or dried
Artichoke hearts
Artichokes
Asparagus
Avocado
Barbecue sauce made with high-fructose corn syrup
Barley
Beets
Biscuits made with wheat, barley, or rye flour
Black beans
Blackberries

Bread made with wheat, barley or rye flour
Breakfast bars
Broccoli
Brussels sprouts
Bulgar wheat
Butter beans
Buttermilk
Cakes made with wheat, barley, or rye flour
Candy, hard or chewy, made with high-fructose corn syrup
Candy, sugar-free, made with "-ol sweeteners"
Cannelloni beans
Cappuccino, unless made with lactose-free milk
Carbonated soft drinks made with high-fructose corn syrup
Carob powder
Cauliflower

Celery
Chamomile tea
Cherries, fresh or dried
Chicory root or extract
Chocolate, white, milk or high% cacao
Cookies made with wheat, barley, or rye flour
Cottage cheese, unless lactose-free
Cough drops, sugar free, made with "-ol" sweetener
Couscous, unless made of rice
Crackers made with wheat, barley, or rye flour flour or grains
Crystalline fructose
Dates
Dry milk solids
Eggnog, unless lactose-free
Enriched flour
Erythritol
Evaporated milk

Fennel leaves

Fennel tea

Fructooligosaccharides (FOS)

Fructose

Fructose solids

Fruit juice concentrates

Fruit punch or fruit juice cocktail made with high-fructose corn syrup

Glycerine

Goat's milk, unless lactose-free

High-fructose corn syrup

Hydrogenated starch hydrolysates

Inulin

Isomalt

Jam or jelly made with high-fructose corn syrup or high-FODMAP fruits

Kamut

Kefir, unless 99% lactose-free

Ketchup made with high-fructose corn syrup

Kidney beans

Lactitol

Lattes, unless made with lactose-free milk

Leeks, white part

Lima beans

Low-carb or "net-carb" bars

Macaroni, white or whole wheat

Maltitol

Mango, fresh or dried

Mannitol

Milkshakes

Milk, unless lactose-free

Molasses

Muffins made with wheat, barley, or rye flour

Mushrooms, fresh or dried

Natural flavorings (in cases which may refer to onions or garlic)

Navy beans

Nectarines

Non-fat dry milk

Onions

Onion powder

Oolong tea

Orzo, white or whole wheat

Pancake syrup made with high fructose corn syrup

Pasta, white or whole wheat

Pesto made with garlic

Peaches, fresh or dried

Pear juice

Pears, fresh or dried

Pinto beans

Pistachios

Plums, fresh or dried

Polydextrose

Preserves made with high-fructose corn syrup or high-FODMAP fruits

Pretzels made with wheat, barley, or rye

Prune juice

Prunes

Pumpkin (U.S.)

Radicchio

Scallions, white part

Semolina flour

Shallots

Snow peas

Sorbitol

Sourdough bread

Soy milk made from whole soy beans

Soy crumbles

Spaghetti, white or whole wheat

Spelt

Spelt bread

Split peas, green, red, or yellow

Sprouted wheat

Sprouted wheat bread

Sugar snap peas

Sweet corn, fresh, frozen, canned

Texturized vegetable protein

Tomato paste

Veggie-burgers

Wasabi paste

Watermelon

Wheat berries

Whey protein concentrate, unless 99% lactose-free

White flour

Whole wheat flour

Xylitol

Yogurt, unless lactose-free

A WEEK OF MENUS

One of the most popular features of *IBS—Free at Last!* is the week of low-FODMAP menus. With that in mind, I created another set of menus for this book which include plenty of recipes. The menus model small, regular meals and snacks, an important part of the FODMAP elimination diet. The meal pattern may need adjusting for IBS patients with small intestinal bacterial overgrowth (SIBO), for which less frequent meals and snacks are often advised. Please note these are merely *sample* menus. You can vary the food choices to suit yourself, referring to the low-FODMAP pantry for inspiration. Some people will need to eat bigger or smaller meals than those in the menus to meet their caloric needs. Also, you are under no obligation to eat a different menu every day for 10 days. If you make a batch of millet muffins, you may choose to repeat that breakfast for several days to use up your muffins. That's perfectly fine. If you have medical conditions besides IBS that impact your nutrition or food choices, please consult a registered dietitian for assistance. Do not eat any food to which you are allergic, even if it appears on these menus.

A few words for vegans, who don't eat any animal products at all. I often get requests for low-FODMAP vegan menus and recipes. Unfortunately, an otherwise perfectly healthy plant-based diet tends to be high in FODMAPs. If you have IBS and you are miserable on a vegan diet with lots of fruits, juices, smoothies, vegetables, avocados, nuts, seeds, and whole grains, then your plant-based diet may be part of the problem. Luckily, tofu which has been pressed and drained (not silken) is low in FODMAPs. Tempeh may also be low in FODMAPs, depending on other ingredients and processing, as is Quorn (plain, mince, or crumbles). Please substitute these protein sources as needed in the menus and recipes in this book. I am including two sample lacto-ovo vegetarian menus (including milk products and eggs) and one sample vegan menu (no animal products at all) that you can use as models for your own meal planning.

As you read through the menus which follow, remember that each food or dish named in the menus should a low-FODMAP version of that food. For example, if "mayonnaise" is listed, it should be a brand that does not contain any high-fructose corn syrup, onions, or garlic. If you need help choosing an appropriate brand, visit me at www.pinterest.com/pcatsos, where you can see pictures of products that meet the requirements for the diet. If you try to purchase any food in the menus ready-made, of course you will be on your own to check the list of ingredients for suitability.

If each word of the recipe title is capitalized, such as Blueberry Millet Muffins, you will find the recipe for that dish in this cookbook.

Day 1

Breakfast
2 scrambled eggs
1 Blueberry Millet Muffin
½ cup Roasted Carrots

Morning Snack
Small handful almonds

Lunch
1 pan-warmed rice tortilla
2 ounces turkey
Lettuce and fresh tomato
2 tablespoons mayonnaise
½ cup grapes

Afternoon Snack
2 strips Beef Jerky
8 cherry tomatoes

Dinner
1 serving Walnut-Encrusted Salmon
Medium baked potato
1 ½ tablespoons sour cream
2 cups raw baby spinach
½ cup slivered red bell pepper
2 tablespoons Lemon Vinaigrette Salad
   Dressing

Beverages
Water, tea or coffee

Day 2

Breakfast
2 fried eggs
1 Corn Griddle Cake
1 teaspoon butter
1 cup lactose-free skim milk
½ ripe banana

Morning Snack
1 hard boiled egg

Lunch
2 fresh Corn Tortillas
3 ounces tuna
1 serving Salsa Ranchera
1 small orange

Afternoon Snack
1 ounce Swiss cheese
8 cherry tomatoes

Dinner
3 ounces grilled turkey burger
1 ounce Cheddar cheese
½ cup brown rice
2 cups mixed salad greens
1 teaspoon olive oil, 1 tablespoon vinegar

Evening Snack
½ cup grapes

Beverages
Water, tea or coffee

Day 3

Breakfast
1 serving Banana Pancakes
1 tablespoon 100% pure maple syrup
1 cup lactose-free skim milk

Morning Snack
½ cup blueberries
½ cup lactose-free cottage cheese

Lunch
1 serving Curried Potato-Tuna Salad
1 cup baby spinach

Afternoon Snack
½ cup of grapes
1 ounce cheddar cheese

Dinner
½ cup Quinoa Pilaf
1 Crispy Baked Pork Chop
1 cup sautéed zucchini and summer squash
1 small orange

Evening Snack
2 tablespoons almonds

Beverages
Water, tea or coffee

Day 4

Breakfast
1 serving Hash Brown Quiche
1 Mini Melon Cup

Morning Snack
½ cup plain oatmeal
½ cup lactose-free skim milk

Lunch
1 Focaccia Roll
2 ounces chicken
1 piece green leaf lettuce
1 tablespoon Brown Maple Mustard
½ cup blueberries
½ cup baby carrots

Afternoon Snack
½ cup lactose-free cottage cheese
1 cup peeled cucumber slices

Dinner
½ cup white or brown rice
1 serving Sizzling Beef Stir-Fry

Evening Snack
1 serving Banana Ice Cream

Beverages
Water, tea or coffee

Day 5

Breakfast
2 slices French Toast
1 tablespoon 100% pure maple syrup
½ cup sliced strawberries
1 cup lactose-free skim milk

Morning Snack
1 wedge Savory Oat Cakes

Lunch
2 cups mixed salad greens
½ cup sliced cucumbers
¼ cup green peas
3 ounces turkey
2 tablespoons Maple Mustard Dressing

Afternoon Snack
½ cup lactose-free cottage cheese
½ cup blueberries

Dinner
4 ounces Grilled Chicken Tidbits
1 serving Lemony Carrot and Pea Salad
1 small orange

Evening Snack
1 serving Rosemary-Scented Rice Crackers
Small handful peanuts

Beverages
Water, tea or coffee

Day 6

Breakfast
1 Zucchini Quinoa Muffin
1 cup lactose-free skim milk

Morning Snack
½ cup strawberries
1 hard-boiled egg

Lunch
1 serving Avgolemono Soup
1 Focaccia Roll
½ cup canned pineapple chunks

Afternoon Snack
1 ounce Cheddar cheese
1 small orange

Dinner
1 serving Shrimp and Grits
½ cup green peas
½ cup red pepper strips

Evening Snack
1 serving Chocolate Pudding

Beverages
Water, tea or coffee

<table>
<tr><td>

Day 7

Breakfast
½ cup sautéed hash-brown potatoes
1 patty Breakfast Sausage
1 egg
½ cup baby spinach
½ cup orange juice

Morning Snack
½ cup grapes
1 ounce string cheese

Lunch
Rice Noodle Bowl for One
½ cup strawberries

Afternoon Snack
½ cup lactose-free yogurt
1 tablespoon 100% pure maple syrup
½ medium red bell pepper, strips

Dinner
1 serving Warm Chicken and Rice Salad
1 serving Asian Cucumber Salad

Evening Snack
½ cup strawberry sorbet

Beverages
Water, tea or coffee

</td><td>

Day 8 (Lacto-Ovo Vegetarian)

Breakfast
1 serving Zucchini Frittata
1 kiwi

Morning Snack
Green Protein Shot

Lunch
1 serving Warm Potato and Green Bean Salad
½ cup lactose-free cottage cheese
8 cherry tomatoes

Afternoon Snack
1 ounce cheddar cheese
½ cup grapes

Dinner
1 cup Quinoa Pilaf
3 ounces Pan Fried Tofu
2 cups mixed salad greens
2 tablespoons Italian Herb Dressing

Evening Snack
1 Chocolate Macaroon

Beverages
Water, tea or coffee

</td></tr>
</table>

Day 9 (Lacto-Ovo Vegetarian)

Breakfast
Morning Muesli Smoothie

Morning Snack
1 Zucchini Quinoa Muffin
1 cup lactose-free milk

Lunch
1 Spinach Quesadilla
½ cup strawberries

Afternoon Snack
½ cup plain lactose-free yogurt
2 teaspoons 100% pure maple syrup
½ medium red bell pepper strips

Dinner
1 serving Risotto with Butternut Squash
½ cup steamed green beans
1 teaspoon butter

Evening Snack
2 Chocolate Macaroons

Beverages
Water, tea or coffee

Day 10 (Vegan)

Breakfast
1 cup cream of buckwheat cereal
½ cup blueberries
½ cup unsweetened rice milk

Morning Snack
1 Corn Griddle Cake
Carrot-Ginger Smoothie

Lunch
1 serving Tempeh Fried Rice
½ cup strawberries

Afternoon Snack
2 tablespoons almond butter
1 brown rice cake

Dinner
1 Quinoa Veggie Burger
2 cups mixed salad greens
2 tablespoons slivered almonds
2 tablespoons Lemon Vinaigrette Salad
    Dressing

Evening Snack
½ cup cantaloupe

Beverages
Water, tea or coffee

SPECIAL OCCASION MENUS

There is no need to apologize to or explain yourself to your guests when you entertain. These menus are so appealing, no one needs to know you are on a special diet unless you choose to tell them. If each word of the recipe title is capitalized, such as Blueberry Millet Muffins, you will find the recipe for that dish in this cookbook. If you try to purchase any food in the menus ready-made, of course you will be on your own to check the list of ingredients for suitability.

Thanksgiving Dinner

Appetizers:
Vegetable platter with Dilly Dip
Warm Spinach Dip with tortilla chips
Roasted, salted macadamia nuts

Main Course:
Roast turkey
Grilled Pork Tenderloin with Pancetta
Barbecued Brisket
Risotto with Butternut Squash

Side Dishes:
Company Mashed Potatoes
Maple Butternut Squash Casserole
Sautéed spinach with slivered almonds
Buttered green peas
Cranberry Orange Relish

Dessert:
Maple Walnut Brittle
Crustless Kabocha Pie

Mother's Day Brunch Buffet

Made-to-order omelets
Home fries
Grilled Pork Tenderloin with Pancetta
Parfaits with Granola and lactose-free yogurt

Spinach salad with strawberries, toasted
    pecans, and Blue Cheese Dressing
Lemony Carrot and Pea Salad
Fresh fruit salad
Magic Coconut Pie

Wedding or Baby Shower

Appetizers:
Hash Brown Quiche
Olive Tapenade with rice crackers
Deviled Eggs
Crab Cakes
Salmon Platter

Salads:
Shrimp and Green Pea Salad
Warm Chicken and Rice Salad
Sliced fresh pineapple, cantaloupe, and
    honeydew melon

Dessert:
Chocolate Macaroons
Lemon Squares

Cocktail Party Buffet

Fresh Thai Spring Rolls
Bacon-Wrapped Water Chestnuts
Potato chips and Roasted Red Pepper Dip
Cheese plate with rice crackers
Assorted olives
Roasted, salted peanuts

Grilled chicken kabobs with Peanut Butter
    Dipping Sauce
Grilled shrimp kabobs with Pineapple Salsa
Carved turkey breast with Focaccia Rolls,
    mayonnaise, and Brown Maple Mustard
Pecan Shortbread Sand Dollars

Valentine's Day

Appetizer:
Green salad with lobster meat and Lemon
    Vinaigrette Salad Dressing

Sides:
Creamy Mashed Potatoes for Two
Roasted Carrots

Main Course:
Walnut-Encrusted Salmon
Grilled filet mignon

Desserts:
Heart-shaped Best Roll-Out Sugar Cookies
Chocolate dipped strawberries
Italian Hot Chocolate

Game Night Buffet

Bacon-Wrapped Water Chestnuts
Tortilla chips with Salsa Ranchera
Seven Layer Salad
Spinach Quesadillas

No-Bean Chili Soup
Warm Potato and Green Bean Salad
Chocolate Pudding

Lobster Bake

Vegetable tray with Roasted Red Pepper Dip
Deviled Eggs
Mom's Fish Chowder
Steamed lobsters with butter

Classic Potato Salad
Lemony Carrot and Pea salad
Fruit salad
Berry-Ricotta Tart

Child's Birthday Party

Grilled hamburgers with Focaccia Rolls
Oven-Fried Potatoes
Mini Melon Cups

Zippy Ketchup
Sundaes with lactose-free ice cream, fresh
     strawberries and Chocolate Syrup

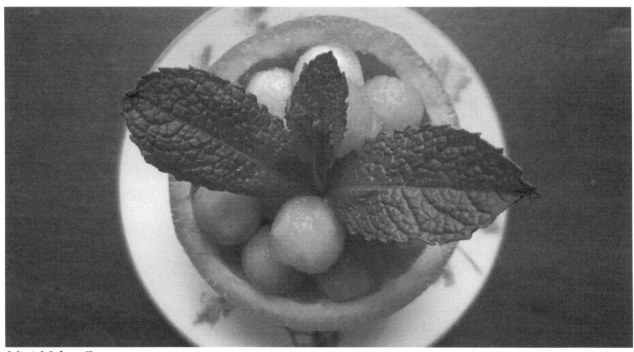

Mini Melon Cup

HOW TO SUCCEED IN THE LOW-FODMAP KITCHEN

Many of your favorite recipes can be easily adapted for use during a low-FODMAP diet. The first step is to identify high-FODMAP ingredients, and to figure out the function of that ingredient in the original recipe. The high-FODMAP ingredient can sometimes be omitted, a much smaller amount can be used to lower the FODMAP load, or a lower-FODMAP ingredient that serves the same function can be substituted.

One important principle of the FODMAP approach is avoiding large loads of FODMAPs at any one meal or snack. How should you handle a recipe that calls for more than one **bold** ingredient from your pantry? Is such a recipe off limits for the FODMAP elimination diet? Not necessarily. I adjusted the recipes in this book so that eating one serving of the recipe as prepared will still keep you within the guidelines of the elimination diet, and you can do the same when you modify your recipes at home. *Please note: if you choose to eat more than one serving of the recipes in this book you may be straying above the recommended portion sizes for certain ingredients.*

These examples illustrate the thought process for modifying recipes to make them lower in FODMAPs:

Salsa with Black Beans (original recipe)	Salsa Ranchero (Low-FODMAP)
1 (8-ounce) can diced tomatoes with roasted garlic and 1 (6-ounce) can tomato paste	1 (14.5-ounce) can Muir Glen organic, fire roasted, diced tomatoes or 4 cups chopped fresh tomatoes
½ cup onions, chopped	1 small bunch scallions, green parts only
2 cloves garlic, minced	2 teaspoons garlic-infused oil
1 cup black beans	1 cup green bell pepper, chopped
1 cup corn kernels	1 cup red bell pepper, chopped
½ cup fresh cilantro, finely chopped	Same
½ teaspoon black pepper, freshly ground	Same
½ teaspoon salt (or to taste)	Same
3 tablespoons fresh lime juice	Same

Starting from the top, replace the seasoned and more concentrated tomato products with the same volume of Muir Glen fire-roasted diced tomatoes or fresh tomatoes. Unless fresh garden tomatoes are in season, go with the Muir Glen—the flavor of the fire-roasted tomatoes is outstanding and will add complexity to the dish. Replace the onions with an equal amount of scallion greens, sliced paper thin. Oil is not a typical salsa ingredient; we are using it here as a vehicle for garlic flavor. Replace the beans and corn with an equal volume of low-FODMAP bell peppers for crunchy texture and color. This salsa tastes fabulous and is now low in FODMAPs.

Macaroni and Cheese (original recipe)	Macaroni and Cheese (low-FODMAP)
8 ounces elbow macaroni	8 ounces elbow macaroni made from corn, quinoa, or rice
1 (12 fluid ounce) can evaporated milk	12 fluid ounces lactose-free milk, 2 tablespoons cornstarch
½ teaspoon salt	Same
½ teaspoon dry mustard	Same
¼ teaspoon black pepper, freshly ground	Same
2 cups Cheddar cheese, shredded	Same
½ cup bread crumbs	½ cup gluten-free bread crumbs or crushed tortilla chips

Use elbow macaroni made of corn (try DeBoles brand) instead of regular macaroni. Evaporated milk has an outrageous amount of lactose in it, so replace it with the same quantity of lactose-free milk. Add 2 tablespoons of corn starch, which will thicken the milk during cooking to a consistency more like that of evaporated milk. Cheddar cheese is low in lactose, so that can stay in the recipe. For a crunchy topping on top of the casserole, replace ordinary bread crumbs with gluten-free bread crumbs. The shorthand in the market place for appropriate bread or bread crumbs is usually "gluten-free," although gluten itself is not a FODMAP. Gluten-free claims can help us identify bread crumbs that don't have wheat, rye, or barley; still, read the label to make sure they don't contain garlic, onions, or other FODMAPs. Another easy option would be to replace the bread crumbs with crushed tortilla chips.

Substitutions for Flavor without FODMAPs

If you lack experience in the kitchen, you may wonder whether recipes will come out right if you change or omit high-FODMAP ingredients. With the exception of baked goods, most recipes will still come out quite well as long as you substitute solids for solids and liquids for liquids. All recipes can have the herbs, spices, and flavorings changed or omitted as needed. Here are a few specific FODMAP-related substitutions you can make as needed. Have courage and give them a try.

If the recipe calls for milk or evaporated milk you can substitute an equal amount of any fluid. The first choice for most people should be lactose-free cow's milk, which is widely available, functions predictably well in recipes, and will make your recipe come out closest to the original in flavor and nutrition. Depending on your caloric needs, you can use skim (non-fat), low-fat, or whole milk. Your choice does not affect the outcome of the recipe technically, though you might prefer the flavor of the whole milk in certain recipes such as chowder. If you can't drink dairy milk, you can substitute rice milk such as Rice Dream or coconut milk beverages like So Delicious. In a few recipes, such as smoothies, you can even use canned coconut milk or coconut cream in place of other fluids if you need to boost calories. These canned coconut products are much more concentrated than coconut milk beverage, so they shouldn't be used to replace milks in other recipes. Trader Joe's coconut milk is a nice product with no additives.

If the recipe calls for yogurt or buttermilk, you can substitute an equal amount of lactose-free yogurt or kefir. Green Valley Organics makes some lovely products. Lifeway kefirs are widely distributed and claim to be 99% lactose-free. In smoothies, you can go even further than that and substitute any other liquid, such as rice milk, coconut milk beverage, and so on. While the texture of the smoothie will certainly change, the smoothie will still be drinkable and tasty.

If the recipe calls for garlic, it may help you to know that the flavor of the garlic is not a problem. You are trying to avoid eating the *flesh* of the garlic, as well as any of the water-soluble fructans that may have leached out into the food. Garlic powder, garlic salt and dehydrated garlic are off limits, as well. If you don't care much for garlic in the first place, by all means omit it. But if you enjoy the flavor of garlic, there are several ways you can get the flavor of the garlic without the FODMAPs. One way is to substitute garlic-infused oil for an equal amount of some other fat or oil in the recipe. For example, if the recipe calls for 2 tablespoons of olive oil, use 2 tablespoons of garlic-infused olive oil instead. You can sometimes add garlic-infused oil just for the flavor, even if the original recipe doesn't call for oil, as we did in the Salsa Ranchero recipe. You can add a teaspoon or two of garlic-infused oil to almost any vegetable, salad, soup, or stew recipe without any negative impact on the outcome. Another way to get the flavor of garlic without the FODMAPs in recipes calling for sautéed, minced garlic is to simply remove the garlic after sautéing it in oil and before adding other ingredients. Snipped garlic chives will contribute convincing garlic flavor, especially in cold recipes such as salad dressings and salsas.

If the recipe calls for onions, use a two-pronged substitution. The flavor of the onions can be provided by the green parts of scallions (green onions), leeks, or chives; an equal amount of a low-FODMAP vegetable can make up for any difference in volume. For example, if a chili recipe calls for 1 cup of chopped onions, you could substitute ¼ cup of scallion greens and ¾ cup of chopped bell peppers. Onion powder, onion salt and dehydrated onion can't be used as substitutes because they contain FODMAPs.

If the recipe calls for other high-FODMAP vegetables, you can substitute an equal amount of any low-FODMAP vegetable. Pay particular attention to whether the vegetables are to be measured raw or after cooking. Some vegetables like spinach cook down so much in cooking that a mismatch here could affect the outcome of the recipe.

If the recipe calls for high-FODMAP fruits, substitute an equal amount of a low-FODMAP fruit. For cold dishes, such as salads, any fruit will do. It is more difficult to replace apples, peaches, and pears in baking, but blueberries, strawberries, rhubarb, and raw cranberries are worth considering.

If the recipe calls for honey or agave syrup, substitute an equal amount of corn syrup such as Karo corn light corn syrup (red label, not the reduced-calorie product), brown rice syrup, or Golden Syrup, either Lyle's brand or homemade from the recipe in this book. If the recipe doesn't require much stickiness from the syrup, substitute 100% pure maple syrup. Maple syrup burns easily, though, so watch your food very carefully as it bakes or cooks. You can also substitute sugar as a sweetener in place of honey or agave, but it is a little more complicated because you have to account for the liquid that honey contributes to the recipe. One cup of honey equals approximately 1 ¼ cups sugar plus ¼ cup liquid. Don't try to substitute stevia for sweeteners in baked goods unless using special recipes designed for the purpose. Stevia extract can easily be used to sweeten smoothies and other cold foods. Just add one drop at a time until the desired level of sweetness is achieved.

If the recipe calls for meat, fish, or poultry, you can use them interchangeably in most recipes. For example, if the recipe calls for a pound of ground pork, you can replace it with an equal amount of ground beef, turkey, or chicken. If the recipe calls for a cup of cooked, diced chicken, you can replace it with a cup of cooked, diced beef, pork, or fish. You can even replace it with a vegetarian form of protein such as a cup of tofu or tempeh if you prefer. Just remember that meat, fish, and poultry shrink about 20% during cooking, so note what is called for in the recipe and plan accordingly. The quantities of meat, fish, and poultry called for in these recipes are raw, unless otherwise specified.

If the recipe calls for pistachios or cashews, you can substitute an equal amount of a low-FODMAP nut. For example, if a recipe calls for ½ cup of chopped pistachios, substitute ½ cup of chopped walnuts or pecans.

If the recipe calls for pasta, choose one made from corn, quinoa or rice instead of one made from wheat or semolina flour.

If the recipe calls for regular bread or bread crumbs, use millet, potato or gluten-free bread, or sourdough-spelt bread. Although a low-FODMAP diet does not necessarily have to be gluten-free, the gluten grains (wheat, barley and rye) are coincidentally high in

FODMAPs. Gluten-free breads are often suitable for a low-FODMAP diet, as long as high-FODMAP ingredients such as inulin, chicory root, or fruit juice concentrates have not been added.

If the recipe calls for flour, think carefully about the function of flour in the recipe. If the flour was to provide a crispy coating for pan-fried or oven-fried food, replace it with an equal amount of rice flour, crushed corn flakes or gluten-free bread crumbs. If the flour was a thickener in a sauce or gravy, replace it with an equal amount of sorghum flour. Corn starch makes a good thickener, too, but use just half as much: replace 2 tablespoons of flour with one tablespoon of corn starch. If flour was the main ingredient in a recipe for a cake, bread, biscuit or cookie recipe it is more difficult to find a worthy substitute. You should probably start by baking recipes that were developed to come out correctly with alternative flours, such as those in this cookbook. Eventually you can experiment with adapting your own recipes, using blends of flours made from alternative grains and starches, ground nuts, or commercial gluten-free flours such as King Arthur's gluten-free all-purpose flour. The less flour in the original recipe, the easier it is to adapt. You will probably have to adjust the amount of liquid in the recipe, and perhaps the baking time, with these alternative flours. Gluten-free recipes are often suitable, since they do not include wheat flour. There are numerous resources available on gluten-free baking, and I recommend you consult them for more on this subject, with one caution: many gluten-free recipes call for the addition of xanthan gum or guar gum to add structure. While these gums are technically not FODMAPs, they are somewhat rapidly fermentable and some people with IBS don't tolerate them in large quantities. Use them with caution, if at all.

If the recipe calls for corn or a corn product, stop for a moment and compare the item called for to your low-FODMAP pantry and label reading food lists. Whole corn kernels (fresh, canned or frozen) are not suitable for the diet because they are naturally high in sorbitol. That's what makes them sweet! Ordinary corn syrup can be used during the elimination phase of the diet even though high-fructose corn syrup is to be avoided. Other corn products, such as cornmeal and corn tortillas are made from corn that is bred to be starchy, rather than sweet, and they are suitable for the elimination phase of the diet. A number of the recipes in the book call for specific types of cornmeal. I've found that the specific grind or type of cornmeal used in a recipe is important to its success. There really is no substitute for either masa harina or masarepa. If you try to use regular corn meal as a substitute for either of these you will be disappointed with the outcome. Even using coarsely ground cornmeal rather than stone ground makes a difference.

Weights, Volumes, and Measures

Now, a little advice about weight, volume, and measures, particularly for those of you who are not experienced cooks. Weights and measures are very important to the success of your recipes. Unless you are a brilliant chef with terrific visual memory, you will not able to estimate a cup of millet flour or a tablespoon of milk with any accuracy, trust me. If you don't already own them, get yourself a nice set of measuring spoons, nesting measuring cups (for solids), and liquid measuring cups in 8, 16, and 24 fluid ounce sizes. Particularly in baking, the proportion of various ingredients must be carefully balanced to get the desired outcome. Make it a rule to follow recipes as closely as possible the first time you make them. If you must make substitutions, follow the guidance in the previous section and try to match the weights, volumes, and measures as closely as possible.

All of the "cups" used in this book refer to United States cups. Metric cups, used in many parts of the world, are slightly larger than United States cups. Cups, tablespoons, and teaspoons are meant to be loosely filled with the food to be measured, and a straight-edge should be scraped across for a level top. If you pack the food in (brown sugar is the only exception), or allow it to heap up over the top of the cup, your measurement will not be accurate, and your recipes will suffer. There are several excellent videos on YouTube about how to weigh and measure ingredients; consider watching them if you've never given this much thought. Here are some common equivalents:

1 ounce (oz) = 28.4 grams (g)

1 pound (lb) = 454 grams (g)

1 fluid ounce (fl oz) = 2 tablespoons (Tb) of liquid = 30 milliliters (ml)

1 quart (qt) = 32 fluid ounces (fl oz) = 960 milliliters (ml)

1 gallon (gal) = 64 fluid ounces (fl oz) = 1.9 liters (L)

1 cup (c): the *weight* of one cup of food depends on what the food is and the size of the cup. One cup of butter weighs much more than one cup of crispy rice cereal, for example.

1 cup (c) = 240 ml. The *volume* of a cup of food does not vary. 1 United States cup is always 240 ml, which is a little smaller than a metric cup (250 ml).

1 tablespoon (T or Tb) = 3 teaspoons (t) = 15 milliliters (ml) ; tablespoons and teaspoons can be used to measure either solids or liquids.

1 teaspoon (t) = 5 milliliters (ml)

½ teaspoon (t) = 2.5 milliliters (ml)

¼ teaspoon (t) = 1.25 milliliters (ml)

Food Language for Global Cooks

People around the world suffer from IBS, and cooks around the world need to prepare food for them. This cookbook was written in the United States, but the terms for some foods and food preparation techniques are different elsewhere. The following is a review of terms used in this book and their foreign equivalents.

Appetizer is also known as starter

Arugula is also known as rocket

Baking soda is also known as bicarbonate of soda

Beet greens are also known as silverbeet

Bell pepper is also known as a sweet pepper or capsicum

Butternut squash is also known as butternut pumpkin

Canned is also known as tinned

Cantaloupe is also known as a rockmelon

Cilantro is also known as coriander leaf

Confectioner's sugar is also known as icing sugar or powdered sugar

Cookies are also known as biscuits

Corn syrup is also known as glucose syrup

Cornmeal is also known as maize flour

Cornstarch is also known as cornflour

Dessert is also known as pudding or afters

Eggplant is also known as aubergine

Endive is also known as chicory or witloof

Garbanzo beans are also known as chickpeas

Granulated sugar is also known as table sugar, white sugar, or sucrose

Green onions are also known as spring onions or scallions

Grilling is also known as barbecuing

Ground meats are also known as minced meats

Ketchup is also known as tomato sauce

Muffin is also known as quick bread

Peanuts are also known as ground nuts

Raisins are also known as sultanas

Raw shrimp are also known as green shrimp

Rice flour is also known as ground rice

Rutabega is also known as swede or turnip

Sausages are also known as bangers

Shredded coconut is also known as desiccated coconut

Shrimp are also known as prawns

Skillet is also known as frying pan

Slice of bacon is also known as rasher of bacon

Sole is also known as bream

Spatula is also known as a fish slice

Stew beef is also known as gravy beef

Stove is also known as range

Stove burner is also known as hob

Summer squash is also known as yellow or crookneck squash

Tuna is also known as tunny

Zucchini is also known as courgette (immature) or marrow (mature)

THE RECIPES

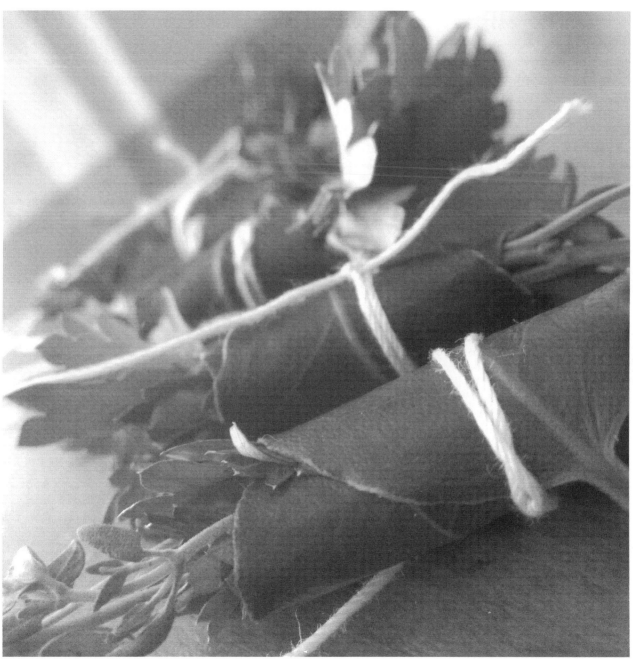

Bouquet Garni

Breads

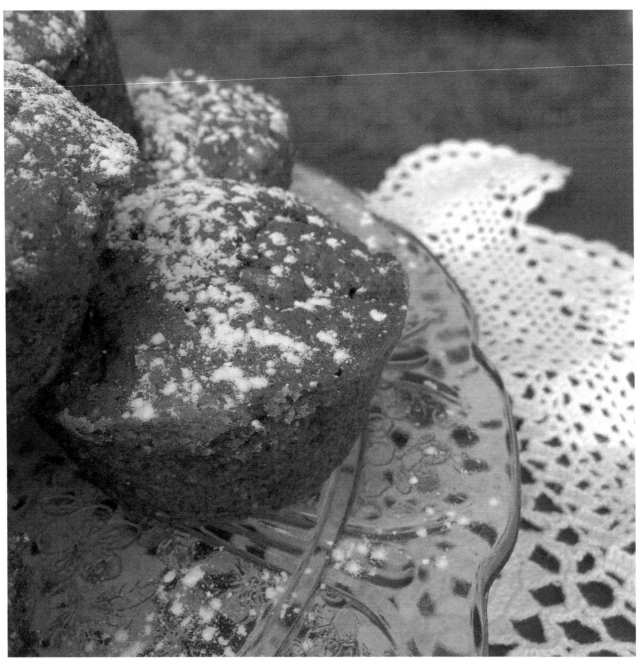

Zucchini Quinoa Muffins

Zucchini Quinoa Muffins

Quinoa flour makes a remarkably light and fluffy muffin. Cornmeal and ground pecans add texture. The familiar aromas of cinnamon and nutmeg make them the perfect after-school treat with a glass of cold milk.

2 large eggs
½ cup granulated sugar
½ cup oil
1 ⅓ cups zucchini, grated
½ cup ground pecans
1 cup quinoa flour
¼ cup stone ground cornmeal
2 teaspoons baking powder
1 teaspoon baking soda
¼ teaspoon salt
¾ teaspoon cinnamon
¼ teaspoon nutmeg

- Preheat the oven to 350° F. Grease a 12-muffin tin with cooking spray and set aside.
- Stir the first four ingredients together in a mixing bowl with a wooden spoon until thoroughly blended.
- Combine remaining ingredients in a separate bowl, then transfer to the zucchini mixture. Stir until dry ingredients are moistened. Divide batter evenly into the prepared muffin tins.
- Bake at 350° F until brown on top and firm to the touch, approximately 20 minutes.
- Serve immediately or cool completely before storing in an airtight container.

Servings: 12

Nutrition Facts

Nutrition (per serving): 180 calories, 9.6g total fat, 250mg sodium, 20.9g carbohydrate, 1.9g fiber, 3.8g protein

Corn Griddle Cakes

Masarepa is a precooked corn flour, so these are almost instantly prepared. Try them with an egg, Cheddar, and red pepper scramble at home or with chili on your next camping trip.

1 cup masarepa
½ teaspoon salt
1 ½ cups water
1 ½ teaspoons butter or oil

- Combine masarepa, salt, and water in a medium-sized bowl. Allow dough to rest for 5 minutes.
- Meanwhile, melt butter (or heat oil) over medium-high heat on a non-stick frying pan or iron skillet. Spoon dough into the pan to create four ½-inch thick cornmeal patties. Sauté until golden brown, approximately 4 minutes on each side. Serve warm.

Servings: 4

Nutrition Facts

Nutrition (per serving): 117 calories, 2.5g total fat, 305mg sodium, 21.7g carbohydrates, 0g fiber, 2.7g protein.

Recipe Tips

This recipe was tested with Goya brand masarepa.
Sprinkle with grated cheese for the last few minutes of cooking, if desired.

Blueberry Millet Muffins

A sweetly crunchy, delicious treat for a special breakfast. Each muffin has four grams of fiber, too.

1 cup plain lactose-free yogurt
2 eggs
⅓ cup oil
⅔ cup light brown sugar, packed
1 ½ cups millet flour
½ cup millet seeds, raw
¼ cup ground chia seeds
1 teaspoon baking powder
¼ teaspoon baking soda
¼ teaspoon salt
⅔ cup fresh or frozen (thawed) blueberries

- Grease a 12-muffin tin with butter.
- Combine the yogurt, eggs, oil, and brown sugar in a medium-sized mixing bowl. Add the remaining ingredients (except blueberries) to the bowl. If the baking soda or baking powder have lumps, sift before adding them. Mix until all dry ingredients are moistened. Do not over-mix. Gently stir in blueberries. Divide batter into the 12 muffin cups in the prepared pan. Sprinkle with extra sugar on top, if desired.
- Preheat oven to 350° F. Allow batter to rest at room temperature while oven is heating up.
- Bake for 20-25 minutes, until golden brown and firm to the touch.
- Cool them for 10 minutes in the muffin pans, then remove them to a wire rack to finish cooling. Store in an airtight container. Muffins freeze well.

Servings: 12

Nutrition Facts

Nutrition (per serving): 265 calories, 9.3g total fat, 146mg sodium, 39.6g carbohydrates, 3.7g fiber, 6.2g protein.

Recipe Tips

This recipe was tested with Filippo Beria Extra Light Tasting olive oil and Bob's Red Mill whole grain millet flour.

Corn Tortillas

No, you don't *have* to make your own corn tortillas, you can buy them ready-made. But if you are looking for some ways to make your low-FODMAP meals extra special, you might enjoy making your own.

1 cup masa harina
½ cup very warm water, approximately

- Place masa harina in a medium mixing bowl. Add warm water to the masa. Use the proportions of masa and water suggested on your bag of masa. Let the dough sit for 5 minutes.
- Work the dough over the bowl for a few minutes, kneading between the palms of your hands. Add a little more water or cornmeal if necessary to get the right consistency. The ball of dough should be smooth on the outside and hold its shape. Divide the dough into 8 pieces; roll each one into a smooth ball. Flatten each ball of dough between 2 sheets of wax paper or between 2 pieces of plastic. Use a tortilla press, skillet, rolling pin, or your hands to flatten the dough into 6-inch circles.
- Heat an ungreased iron skillet over high heat. Cook tortillas, one at a time, for about 30 seconds to a minute on each side. Tortillas should be golden brown and forming little air pockets.
- Press down on the flipped tortilla with a wadded up paper towel, to encourage browning and air pocketing.

- Wrap tortillas in a clean dish towel to stay warm until serving.

    Servings: 8

Nutrition Facts

Nutrition (per serving): 52 calories, <1g total fat, 1mg sodium, 10.9g carbohydrates, 0g fiber, 1.3g protein.

Recipe Tips

Masa harina is a cornmeal product that has been processed in a very specific way for making tortillas. Do not attempt to substitute other forms of cornmeal.

An iron skillet is the perfect pan for cooking corn tortillas; it will not be damaged between tortillas by being empty at high heat..

Cut open a gallon-sized freezer bag and you will have the perfect wrapper for rolling your tortillas in.

There is an art to making tortillas. Check YouTube for demonstration of the technique.

Focaccia Rolls

The gluten added to these rolls produces a crustier, chewier roll than would otherwise be possible. Adapted from a recipe contributed by Diane.

1 tablespoon active dry yeast (1 packet)
1 ⅓ cups very warm water (90-105 ° F)
2 tablespoons granulated sugar
3 tablespoons olive oil, divided
1 large egg
2 ⅓ cups oat flour
⅔ cup tapioca flour
⅓ cup vital wheat gluten
1 teaspoon salt, divided
3 tablespoons cornmeal
1 tablespoon fresh rosemary, crushed, or 2 teaspoons dried

- Combine dry yeast, very warm (not hot) water, and sugar in a small bowl. Observe for a few minutes to make sure there is some yeast activity—usually it looks like fluffy, tan blobs rising to the top of the water. Add the egg and 2 tablespoons olive oil to the yeast mixture.
- Combine oat flour, tapioca flour, vital wheat gluten, and ¾ teaspoon salt in a large mixing bowl. Pour the yeast mixture into the bowl. Mix with an electric mixer for 3 minutes or so to develop the gluten. Add the crushed rosemary just before the end of mixing. Dough will be wet and sticky. Cover with plastic wrap and leave in a warm place to rise until it has doubled, about 1 ½ hours.
- Preheat oven to 450° F, and sprinkle the cornmeal on the ungreased cookie tray.
- Divide the cookie dough into 10 balls and place on the cookie tray. Brush the rolls with the remaining olive oil using a pastry brush, sprinkle with remaining salt and a little additional rosemary.
- Bake for 25 minutes. Rolls are done when uniformly medium brown.
- Remove tray from the oven. Transfer rolls to a wire rack. Cool completely before cutting for best results.

    Servings: 10

Nutrition Facts

Nutrition (per serving): 188 calories, 6g total fat, 250mg sodium, 27.3g carbohydrates, 2.6g fiber, 6.8g protein.

Recipe Tips

Very warm water can be prepared by heating 1 ⅓ cups cold water in the microwave for 45 seconds.

When measuring dry ingredients such as flour for baking, precision is important. First, stir the flour. Spoon it lightly into the measuring cup or spoon, then run a flat blade across the top. Make sure the flour is neither packed down nor "heaping".

Rosemary-Scented Rice Crackers

Delicious as is or with a bit of dip, spread, or cheese. Thank you, Mary Ann, for sharing this recipe.

> ½ cup brown rice flour
> 1 teaspoon olive oil
> ½ teaspoon sea salt
> ¼ teaspoon fresh rosemary, minced, or more to taste
> ¼ cup water

- Preheat oven to 425° F.
- Combine all ingredients in a medium-sized mixing bowl until thoroughly blended.
- Pat the dough out on an ungreased cookie sheet using a spoon, then your fingers, until it is about $\frac{1}{16}$ -inch thick. Score with a knife into squares or rectangles, if desired.
- Bake for 10 minutes, then turn oven off and allow crackers to cook with the oven door closed for another 10 minutes.
- Using a thin metal spatula, remove crackers from the cookie sheet and store in an airtight container. These keep well for up to a week.

> Servings: 6

Nutrition Facts

Nutrition (per serving): 54 calories, 1.1g total fat, 158mg sodium, 10.1g carbohydrates, <1g fiber, <1g protein.

Old-Fashioned Spoon Bread

Spoon bread is a Southern comfort food, buttery and delicious when eaten warm from the oven.

> ¾ cup stone ground cornmeal
> ½ teaspoon salt
> 1 cup water
> 3 tablespoons butter
> 1 tablespoon granulated sugar
> 1 cup lactose-free milk
> 2 large eggs, beaten
> 2 teaspoons baking powder

- Preheat the oven to 350° F. Generously butter an 8" by 8" glass baking dish.
- Combine cornmeal, salt, sugar, and water in a medium saucepan. Stir constantly over medium heat until the mixture comes to a boil. Remove from heat. Stir in sugar and butter until butter is melted. Stir in cold milk and blend with a whisk until smooth. Add eggs and baking powder and whisk until smooth.
- Transfer the mixture to the baking dish and bake at 350° F for about 40 minutes, until golden brown on edges and slightly puffy in the middle.
- Serve warm.

> Servings: 9

Nutrition Facts

Nutrition (per serving): 102 calories, 5.3g total fat, 296mg sodium, 10.9g carbohydrates, <1g fiber, 3.2g protein.

Recipe Tips

This recipe was tested with Bob's Red Mill stone ground cornmeal and it came out perfectly. I've found that using that the type and grind of cornmeal specified in recipes is critical to their success.

Savory Oat Cakes

Somehow these taste like Cheeze-Its.

1 cup quick cooking oats
1 cup oat flour
¼ teaspoon sea salt
¼ teaspoon dry mustard
¼ cup unsalted butter
1 cup sharp Cheddar cheese, shredded
½ cup warm water

- Preheat oven to 400° F. Grease a large cookie sheet with butter and set aside.
- Stir oats, oat flour, sea salt, and mustard together in medium-sized mixing bowl. Cut in butter, using pastry cutter, until the mixture has a coarse, sandy texture. Stir in shredded cheese. Add water; mix with a fork until stiff dough forms. Using clean hands, knead the dough in the bowl until all crumbs are incorporated into the dough.
- Divide dough in two and form flattened disks of dough. Press the dough out into circles about ¼-inch thick on the cookie tray. Circles should be approximately 7 inches in diameter. Cut each circle into 8 wedges.
- Bake for 20 minutes, then turn off the oven and let cool with the oven door closed for another 20 minutes.
- Remove from cookie sheets, cool slightly and serve the same day if you like them crispy. Store leftovers in an airtight container.

Servings: 16

Nutrition Facts

Nutrition (per serving): 122 calories, 6.6g total fat, 75mg sodium, 11.5g carbohydrates, 1.5g fiber, 4.5g protein.

"Bread" Crumbs

You can buy so-called bread crumbs that are low in FODMAPs, but they are expensive and come in packages that may be too large for your needs. Try this recipe the next time you need a small batch of crumbs to bread chicken or to sprinkle on top of a casserole.

⅓ cup raw pecan pieces
⅓ cup crispy rice cereal
⅓ cup corn flakes
⅛ teaspoon sea salt
⅛ teaspoon black pepper, freshly ground

- Toast pecans briefly over medium heat in an ungreased heavy skillet, stirring constantly until slightly browned.
- Place all ingredients in the bowl of a blender. Use a pulsing action to grind ingredients to the consistency of coarse grains of sand.
- Use immediately or store, covered, in the refrigerator.

Servings: 8

Nutrition Facts

Nutrition (per serving): 40 calories, 3.3g total fat, 51mg sodium, 26.4 carbohydrates, .5g fiber, .6g protein.

Recipe Tips

Make these crumbs "Italian style" by adding Italian seasoning to taste. Check the label to make sure the seasoning blend contains green herbs only.

ab

Breakfast Dishes

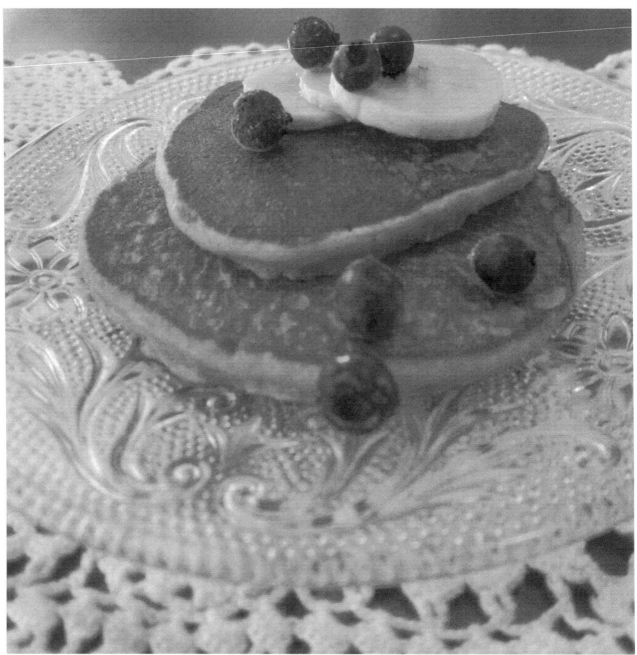

Banana Pancakes; photo by Christine Beecher

Banana Pancakes

These make a special breakfast, served steaming hot with real butter and maple syrup.

> ½ **cup rolled oats**
> ½ **c sorghum flour**
> **1 teaspoon baking powder**
> **1 cup lactose-free cottage cheese**
> **3 large eggs**
> **1 large banana**
> **1 teaspoon butter**

- Combine all ingredients in a blender until smooth. Add lactose-free milk if necessary for pouring consistency.
- Use additional butter or cooking spray to lightly grease a non-stick griddle or skillet.
  Heat the skillet over medium-low heat until butter is fragrant. Pour pancake batter onto the hot griddle. Turn with spatula when edges are dry and top is starting to firm up. Pancake is done when the middle puffs up.
- Serve immediately or keep warm in a 200°F oven on an oven-proof plate until serving.

> Servings: 4

Nutrition Facts

Nutrition (per serving): 211 calories, 6.7g total fat, 308mg sodium, 23.6g carbohydrates, 3.3g fiber, 14.8g protein.

Breakfast Sausage

Put breakfast sausage back on the menu with this freshly made version.

> **2 pounds ground pork**
> **4 teaspoons ground sage**
> **1 ½ teaspoons salt**
> **1 teaspoon ground black pepper**
> ½ **teaspoon crushed red pepper flakes (optional)**
> **1 tablespoon 100% pure maple syrup**

- Combine all ingredients in a large mixing bowl using a wooden spoon or clean hands.
- Portion meat with a ¼ cup measure and flatten into ⅓-inch thick patties.
- Warm a little olive oil in a skillet over medium heat if your ground pork is very lean; otherwise, skip this step. Fry patties in a skillet over medium heat for 5-6 minutes on each side, until browned and no longer pink in the center.
- Serve immediately or freeze to reheat at a later date.

> Servings: 14, 1 patty each

Nutrition Facts

Nutrition (per serving): 174 calories, 13.8g total fat, 285mg sodium, <1g carbohydrates, <1g fiber, 11g protein.

Buckwheat Pancakes

These are delicious. I enjoy wheat-free cooking with traditional ingredients, rather than using mixes that try to imitate conventional foods. Buckwheat pancakes are an old favorite.

> **1 large egg slightly beaten**
> **1 cup lactose-free milk**
> **1 tablespoon cider vinegar**
> **1 cup buckwheat flour**
> **2 tablespoons brown sugar, packed**
> **¾ teaspoon baking soda**
> **½ teaspoon salt**
> **½ teaspoon ground cinnamon**
> **¼ teaspoon ground nutmeg**

- In a medium-sized bowl, mix together the egg, milk, and vinegar. Add the dry ingredients and stir to mix until well combined.
- Heat a large non-stick skillet over medium heat. Lightly grease with butter or oil.
- Pour pancake batter onto the skillet and cook 3-4 minutes until bubbles form all over the pancake and edges are slightly dry. Turn and cook the second side until golden brown and cooked through, 2-3 minutes.
- Serve warm with 100% pure maple syrup, butter, low-FODMAP jam, or fruit.

> Servings: 4

Nutrition Facts

Nutrition (per serving): 168 calories, 2.3g total fat, 575mg sodium, 31.4g carbohydrates, 3.2g fiber, 7.5g protein.

French Toast

This recipe makes low-FODMAP bread shine. Make extra to reheat on busy weekday mornings.

> **4 large eggs**
> **½ cup lactose-free milk**
> **1 teaspoon vanilla**
> **8 slices sourdough-spelt or gluten-free bread**
> **1 teaspoon cinnamon**
> **1 tablespoon butter**

- Combine the eggs, milk, and vanilla in a 9" by 13" baking dish. Soak the slices of bread in the egg and milk mixture. Sprinkle liberally with cinnamon.
- Melt part of the butter over medium heat in a large non-stick pan or griddle. When the butter is bubbling, place a single layer of bread slices in the pan. If there is a little extra egg mixture, pour it into the center of each bread slice in the pan. Cook until the bottom of the toast is golden brown, approximately 2-3 minutes. Flip over and cook the other side until golden brown. Center of toast should puff up slightly when done. Repeat with remaining slices of bread.
- Serve warm with 100% pure maple syrup, butter, low-FODMAP jam, or fruit.

> Servings: 4

Nutrition Facts

Nutrition (per serving): 268 calories, 10.1g total fat, 415mg sodium, 30.9g carbohydrates, 1.9g fiber, 12.4g protein.

Granola

It just feels good to eat this granola. Due to its moderate FODMAP content, think of it as a "topping" for lactose-free yogurt or ice cream, not a cereal to eat by the bowlful.

3 cups rolled oats
1 cup millet seeds, raw
½ cup walnut pieces
½ cup chia seeds
½ cup pecans, chopped
½ cup pumpkin seeds
¼ cup oil
⅓ cup 100% pure maple syrup
1 teaspoon vanilla
⅛ teaspoon nutmeg
½ teaspoon cinnamon

- Preheat oven to 325° F.
- Measure oats, millet, nuts, and seeds into a large mixing bowl.
- Combine oil, maple syrup, vanilla, cinnamon, and nutmeg in a glass measuring cup. Pour over the oat mixture, and stir to coat. Transfer the mixture into an ungreased 9" by 13" baking dish.
- Bake for approximately 1 hour, stirring every 15 minutes. Watch closely to make sure it doesn't burn.
- Remove from the oven and allow to cool thoroughly before storing in an airtight container.

Servings: 32

Nutrition Facts

Nutrition (per serving): 104 calories, 6.1g total fat, 6mg sodium, 11.6g carbohydrates, 1.5g fiber, 2.5g protein.

Hash Brown Quiche

This versatile recipe will serve 10 for brunch and reheats well for breakfast at the office.

32 ounces frozen hash brown potatoes, thawed
2 cups cooked ham, diced (optional)
2 cups shredded Cheddar cheese
3 scallions, green part only, thinly sliced
1 red bell pepper, chopped
1 cup lactose-free milk
10 large eggs, lightly beaten
½ teaspoon black pepper, freshly ground

- Preheat oven to 425° F. Grease a 9" by 13" pan with butter on the bottom and sides.
- Press thawed potatoes into the pan.
- Bake for 25 minutes at 425° F, then remove from the oven and turn the heat down to 350° F.
- Spread ham, onion, red pepper, and cheese evenly across hot potatoes.
- Combine milk, egg, and black pepper in a large measuring cup or bowl and pour over other ingredients.
- Bake at 350° F for 30-40 more minutes or until cheese is golden brown and a knife inserted in the center of the casserole comes out clean.

Servings: 10

Nutrition Facts

Nutrition (per serving): 295 calories, 14.6g total fat, 613mg sodium, 19.3g carbohydrates, 1.6g fiber, 21.9g protein.

Beverages

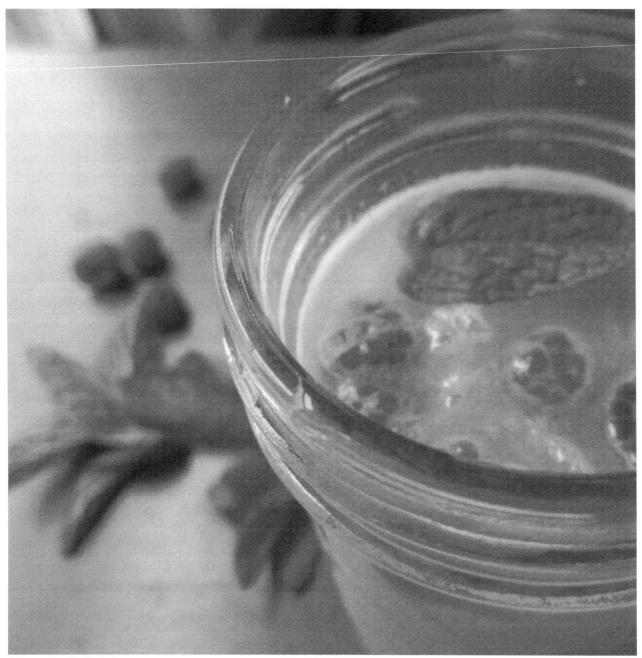

Fizzy Fruit Drink

Do you consider smoothies and juices the healthiest part of your diet? Unfortunately, with the wrong protein powder and too much fruit, they can be FODMAP bombs. Often consumed at breakfast, the poorly-absorbed fructose, sugar alcohols, and lactose in smoothies hit your large intestine by lunchtime and can contribute to afternoon and evening GI distress. The beverage recipes in this book are gut-friendly because they use low-FODMAP ingredients and because they limit fruit to ½ cup per serving.

Smoothies are very versatile and can handle a lot of variation to meet your personal needs and preferences. In each of the following recipes, any liquid can be used in place of the one called for. For example, if you need to gain weight, you can use canned coconut milk for the liquid and frozen cubes of coconut cream instead of regular ice cubes. If you are a vegan, you can use rice, coconut milk beverage, or coconut water instead of cow's milk, yogurt or kefir. Stay away from most soy milk and soy yogurts, though. In the United States they are usually high in FODMAPs. Cultured coconut milk (similar to yogurt) and frozen desserts made from coconut milk tend to have high-FODMAP ingredients such as inulin and chicory root added, so avoid them too.

Protein powders are popular smoothie ingredients, though not a necessary part of the diet for most people. I find that 99% lactose-free whey protein powders mix most smoothly into blender drinks. Ingredients to avoid in protein powders include whey protein concentrate (unless accompanied by a 99% lactose-free claim), fructose (common in chocolate protein powders), and added fibers. Vegans can substitute rice protein powder as needed in any smoothie. Avoid protein powders from soy, hemp, peas, and other sources until we know more about their FODMAP content.

Fizzy Fruit Sparkler

Small servings of fruit juice are best for people with IBS, so this refreshing fizzy drink is a great fit.
- **⅓ cup crushed ice**
- **⅓ cup orange juice**
- **⅓ cup orange-flavored sparkling water**
- **6 frozen red raspberries**
- **1 mint leaf**

• Measure the crushed ice into an 8-10 fluid ounce glass. Add the orange juice and sparkling water. Top with frozen berries, garnish with mint leaf, and serve immediately.

Servings: 1

Nutrition Facts

Nutrition (per serving): 66 calories, <1g total fat, 5mg sodium, 16.5g carbohydrates, 1.5g fiber, .8g protein

Berry Banana Smoothie

This smooth and creamy combination is a protein-packed breakfast or snack. It is low-calorie as written, but can easily be modified for those who need to gain weight by using frozen coconut cream instead of ice cubes.

½ cup plain lactose-free yogurt
½ cup coconut water
¼ cup blueberries, raspberries, or strawberries
¼ banana, frozen
1 serving protein powder
2 ice cubes
2 drops liquid stevia (optional)

- Place ingredients in the bowl of a blender in the order listed. Blend on high until a uniform consistency is reached.
- Serve immediately.

Servings: 1

Nutrition Facts

Nutrition (per serving): 181 calories, 2.3g total fat, 233mg sodium, 25.9g carbohydrates, 4.3g fiber, 14.9g protein.

Recipe Tips

Plan ahead for this smoothie by peeling, quartering, and freezing ripe bananas with the pieces spread out in a freezer bag. When it's smoothie time, just pull a piece out of the bag and return the rest to the freezer.
For an extra 175 calories, use 2 cubes of frozen coconut cream instead of ice cubes. Canned coconut cream can be frozen ahead of time in ice cube trays and stored in a freezer bag.
This recipe was tested with Green Valley lactose-free plain yogurt and Dr. Sears Zone protein powder.

Morning Muesli Smoothie

Breakfast to go, featuring kefir, a fermented milk beverage which contains a wide range of beneficial probiotics. This smoothie is a small, well-balanced meal.

¼ cup water
¾ cup plain lactose-free kefir
2 tablespoons quick oats
1 ½ teaspoons whole or ground chia seeds
¼ cup frozen blueberries
⅛ teaspoon cinnamon
2 ice cubes
2 drops stevia extract (optional)

- Place all ingredients in the bowl of a blender in the order listed.
- Blend on high until a uniform consistency is reached.
- Serve immediately or bring to work in a thermos.

Servings: 1

Nutrition Facts

Nutrition (per serving): 190 calories, 4.8g total fat, 131mg sodium, 25.9g carbohydrates, 3.3g fiber, 11.7g protein.

Carrot Lemonade Smoothie

Smoothies, unlike juices, don't have fiber strained out. If you are looking for low-FODMAP vitamins in a liquid form, vegetable smoothies like this one can help.

½ cup ice water
1 medium carrot, peeled and quartered
1 small lemon, peeled
1 ½ tablespoons 100% pure maple syrup
3 ice cubes

• Put all ingredients in the bowl of a blender in the order listed. Blend on high until the desired consistency is reached. If you are using a high speed blender, the carrots can be completely liquified.
• Serve immediately.

Servings: 1

Nutrition Facts

Nutrition (per serving): 118 calories, <1g total fat, 49mg sodium, 31.1g carbohydrates, 1.9g fiber, <1g protein.

Carrot-Ginger Smoothie

This recipe makes eating more fruits and vegetables easy and delicious.

½ cup coconut water
1 medium orange, peeled
1 large carrot, peeled and quartered
¼-inch piece of ginger root, peeled, or more to taste
3 coconut water ice cubes

• Place all ingredients in the bowl of a blender in the order listed. Blend on high until a uniform consistency is reached.
• Serve immediately

Servings: 1

Nutrition Facts

Nutrition (per serving): 150 calories, <1g total fat, 277mg sodium, 34.7g carbohydrates, 7.4g fiber, 3.8g protein.

Rice Milk

A high-speed blender (like a Vitamix) is a must for this recipe. Treat yourself to a fresh batch of rice milk each day.

¼ cup cooked brown short grain rice, cooled to room temperature
1 cup cold water
1 teaspoon 100% pure maple syrup or a drop of stevia

• Add ingredients to the bowl of a high speed blender. Blend on high for 2 minutes.
• Transfer to a glass jar, cover, and chill until serving. Use within 24 hours.

Servings: 1

Nutrition Facts

Nutrition (per serving): 99 calories, <1g total fat, 7mg sodium, 23.7g carbohydrates, 1.4g fiber, 1.4g protein.

Green Protein Shot

Add some extra protein, fiber and vitamin A to your breakfast with one serving of this green smoothie. Bring the other serving to work in a small thermos for a mid-morning boost.

    ½ cup water
    1 cup plain, lactose-free yogurt
    1 medium orange, peeled
    ½ medium banana, peeled
    2 cups baby kale or spinach
    1 serving protein powder
    6 ice cubes

- Place ingredients in the bowl of a blender in the order listed. Blend on high until a uniform consistency is reached.
- Serve immediately.

    Servings: 2

Nutrition Facts

Nutrition (per serving): 185 calories, 2.5g total fat, 148mg sodium, 30.3g carbohydrates, 4.2g fiber, 13.1g protein.

Greensleeves Smoothie

This smoothie ups your intake of electrolytes and antioxidants in a most delicious way.

    ½ cup coconut water
    1 Roma tomato, quartered
    ½ lime, peeled
    1 cup baby kale or spinach
    8 sprigs parsley
    1 medium carrot, peeled and quartered
    3 coconut water ice cubes

- Place ingredients in the bowl of a blender in the order listed. Blend on high until a uniform consistency is reached.
- Serve immediately.

    Servings: 1

Nutrition Facts

Nutrition (per serving): 126 calories, 1.3g total fat, 334mg sodium, 26.9g carbohydrates, 6.9g fiber, 5.3g protein.

Vegan Green Velvet Smoothie

For extra calories use canned coconut milk or cream instead of coconut milk beverage.

1 cup rice or coconut milk beverage, unsweetened
1 cup baby kale or spinach
½ cup green grapes
1 serving rice protein powder
2 drops stevia
3 coconut water ice cubes

- Place all ingredients in the bowl of a blender in the order listed. Blend on high until a uniform consistency is reached.
- Serve immediately.

Servings: 1

Nutrition Facts

Nutrition (per serving): 276 calories, 3.7g total fat, 189mg sodium, 50.3g carbohydrates, 3.2g fiber, 14.6g protein.

Italian Hot Chocolate

The secret ingredient for Italian-style hot chocolate is cornstarch, which makes it thicker and creamier than regular hot chocolate.

2 tablespoons granulated sugar
2 tablespoons cocoa powder
1 ½ teaspoons cornstarch
pinch of salt
1 ½ cups lactose-free milk
¼ teaspoon vanilla extract

- Combine the dry ingredients in a 2-cup microwave-safe container such as a glass measuring cup. Add milk up to the 1 ½-cup mark, then stir in vanilla extract.
- Microwave on high in one minute intervals for three minutes, stirring after each. Stop just before it comes to a boil.
- Pour into two small teacups and serve warm. Top with whipped cream if desired.

Servings: 2

Nutrition Facts

Nutrition (per serving): 146 calories, 4.2g total fat, 154mg sodium, 22.1g carbohydrates, 1.47g fiber, 6.8g protein

Appetizers

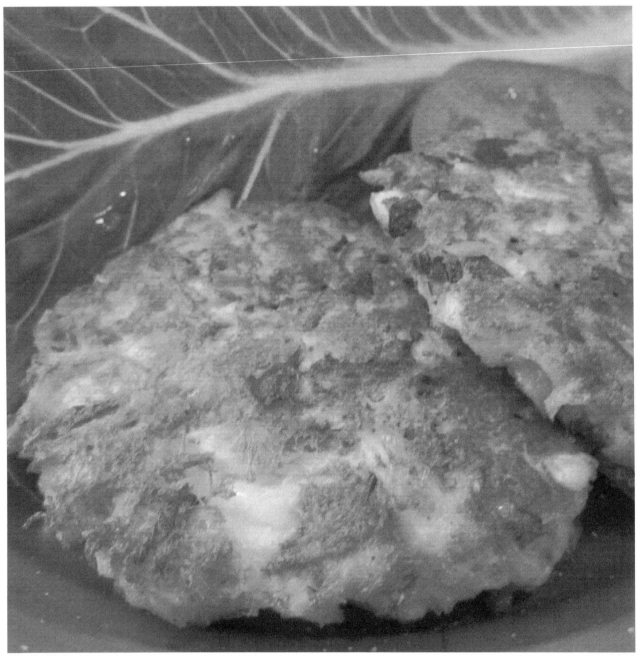

Crab Cakes

Crab Cakes

Sometimes less is more. There are few distractions from the delicate flavor of crab meat in this recipe.

1 tablespoon butter
½ cup fennel bulb, finely chopped
¼ cup parsley, finely chopped
½ teaspoon salt
½ teaspoon black pepper, freshly ground
12 ounces lump crab meat
2 tablespoons wheat-free bread crumbs
1 tablespoon real mayonnaise
1 teaspoon whole grain mustard
2 large eggs, well beaten
2 tablespoons garlic-infused extra virgin olive oil

- Melt butter in a large non-stick frying pan or iron skillet over medium heat. Add fennel bulb and parsley, and cook over medium-low heat until fennel is tender, about 10 minutes, stirring occasionally. Set aside to cool.
- Meanwhile, combine the remaining ingredients (except oil) in a medium-sized mixing bowl. Add cooled fennel mixture.
- Heat the oil over medium-high heat in the frying pan. Drop crab mixture in bite-size spoonfuls into the hot oil and shape into patties. Fry for 4-5 minutes on each size, until crispy and browned.
- Serve on a bed of lettuce. Garnish with a colorful spoonful of Salsa Ranchera, if desired.

Servings: 8

Nutrition Facts

Nutrition (per serving): 122 calories, 8.0g total fat, 237mg sodium, 2.4g carbohydrates, <1g fiber, 9.7g protein.

Recipe Tips

Buy lump crab meat already picked in the refrigerated seafood section of your grocery store. This recipe was tested with North Coast Seafood Culinary Reserve claw crab meat. Don't waste your time using cheap canned crab meat from the grocery aisle.
Fennel has a mild flavor and a crispy texture, like celery.

Dilly Dip

Serve this as a dip for vegetables or corn chips, or as a sauce on chicken or lamb kabobs.

1 cup plain, lactose-free, low-fat yogurt
½ cup cucumber peeled, seeded and cut into ¼-inch cubes
2 tablespoons minced fresh dill or 1 tablespoon dried dill
½ teaspoon sweet, smoked paprika
2 tablespoons fresh lemon juice
½ teaspoon salt
¼ teaspoon black pepper, freshly ground

- Combine ingredients in a small mixing bowl. Adjust seasonings to taste.
- Cover and chill until serving.

Servings: 10

Nutrition Facts

Nutrition (per serving): 19 calories, <1g total fat, 134mg sodium, 2.5g carbohydrates, <1g fiber, 1.4g protein.

Bacon-Wrapped Water Chestnuts

Watch these disappear at your next party.

1 (16 ounce) can whole water chestnuts, drained
⅓ cup rice wine vinegar
1 teaspoon brown sugar
¾ pound bacon, thinly sliced

- Cut the largest water chestnuts in half so that all pieces are a uniform size. Combine the rice wine vinegar and brown sugar in a medium-sized bowl. Add the water chestnuts and marinate for at least 1 hour. Drain.
- Preheat the oven to 400° F.
- Cut the bacon strips in half, so that each strip is about 4 inches long. Wrap each water chestnut with half a strip of bacon, and secure with a plain wooden toothpick. Place the wrapped water chestnuts on a baking sheet so that they are not touching each other.
- Bake for 15 minutes, turn over and bake for another 10 minutes or until bacon is crispy.
- Transfer water chestnuts to clean paper towels briefly to allow grease to drain, then serve immediately.

Servings: 28

Nutrition Facts

Nutrition (per serving): 26 calories, 1.4g total fat, 36mg sodium, 1.8g carbohydrates, <1g fiber, 1.4g protein.

Recipe Tips

This recipe was tested with Applegate Naturals bacon and Geisha whole water chestnuts.

Deviled Eggs

Deviled eggs are an old-fashioned treat that still taste as good as ever. They are inexpensive, too. Make a batch for your next backyard barbecue or tailgate party.

12 large eggs
¼ cup mayonnaise
2 teaspoons whole grain mustard

- Place eggs in a 4-quart saucepan and cover them with cold water. Bring water to a rolling boil. Turn off heat, and let eggs sit in boiled water for 20 minutes. Drain off hot water, and rinse eggs several times in cold water.
- Fill egg pan with cold water. Gently squeeze each egg until the shell is crushed enough to let water seep in. Let the eggs sit in cold water for a few minutes, then remove and discard shells.
- Halve each egg lengthwise with a sharp knife. Collect egg yolks in a bowl and set egg whites aside.
- Mash egg yolks, mayonnaise, and mustard together until very smooth. Season with salt and pepper to taste. Add more mayonnaise or mustard to taste. Fill the egg white halves with spoonfuls of egg yolk mixture. If desired, garnish the eggs with a sprinkling of paprika or little dabs of mustard.
- Cover and chill until serving.

Servings: 12

Nutrition Facts

Nutrition (per serving): 97 calories, 7g total fat, 106mg sodium, 1.8g carbohydrates, <1g fiber, 6.4g protein.

Beef Jerky

This beef jerky is a nice portable snack. It may take a little practice to recognize when the jerky is done; otherwise this is a very easy recipe.

> **2 pounds lean beef**
> **⅓ cup reduced-sodium soy sauce**
> **1 teaspoon ground black pepper**
> **1 tablespoon 100% pure maple syrup**
> **2 teaspoons hot pepper sauce (optional)**

- Trim off all visible fat; slice beef into uniform, thin (¼-inch) slices, across the grain. Place the beef strips in a gallon zipper-top freezer bag.
- Combine the remaining ingredients in a small bowl, then pour over the beef in the bag. Squeeze out excess air, zip it, and manipulate the bag to coat the beef on all sides with the marinade. Place the bag in refrigerator overnight to marinate.
- The next day, line 2 cookie sheets with aluminum foil; place wire racks on the cookie sheets. Arrange the beef slices in a single layer on the wire racks. Place cookie sheets in a cold oven. Set the oven to 160° F and begin to heat it up.
- Bake with the door closed until 5 minutes after the oven comes up to temperature. Prop the oven door open slightly for remainder of oven time. Bake for 4 or more hours until beef strips are dry to the touch but still pliable.
- Store tightly covered in the refrigerator for up to 2 weeks.

> Servings: 32

Nutrition Facts

Nutrition (per serving): 84 calories, 6.5g total fat, 110mg sodium, <1g carbohydrates, <1g fiber, 5.2g protein.

Recipe Tips

Freeze the beef for an hour before slicing to make it easier to handle.

Kalamata Tapenade

This party-sized, gourmet dip tastes great with rice crackers, tortilla chips, or carrot sticks.

> **1 pound Kalamata olives, pitted, about 2 ½ cups**
> **juice of one lemon**
> **⅓ cup fresh parsley, chopped**
> **⅓ cup garlic-infused extra virgin olive oil**
> **¼ teaspoon black pepper, freshly ground**

- Pulse all the ingredients in a food processor or large blender until uniform, coarse, small pieces are produced.
- Chill for up to 24 hours before serving.

> Servings: 24

Nutrition Facts

Nutrition (per serving): 55 calories, 5.8g total fat, 168mg sodium, <1g carbohydrates, <1g fiber, <1g protein.

Recipe Tips

Other types of olives can be substituted for the Kalamatas if desired

Fresh Thai Spring Rolls

Spring roll wrappers are surprisingly easy to work with after you get the hang of it. Gather the gang around and a have a spring rolling party.

2 cups lettuce, shredded
1 bunch basil, leaves only
1 bunch cilantro, leaves only
2 medium carrots, peeled and shredded
1 medium cucumber, peeled, and cut into match sticks
8 large shrimp, peeled, cooked, deveined, and cut in half lengthwise
4 ounces rice sticks or vermicelli
16 spring roll wrappers (rice paper)

• Prepare the rice sticks according to package directions, drain, and set aside. If directions are unclear, cover rice sticks with boiling water and allow them to soften for 5-8 minutes. Do not overcook.
• Set up your work area with a large empty plate in front of you, a large bowl of very warm water on hand, and all ingredients nearby.
• Soak one rice paper at a time in the warm water for about 30 seconds, until it begins to soften up but is not too limp. The rice paper circle should be just short of collapsing when you remove it from the water. Spread the wet rice paper out on the plate.
• Place some of the vegetables, shrimp, and rice stick in a rectangle-shaped area toward the front of the circular rice paper. (Picture a stick of butter placed off-center on a round plate.) Fold the front of the rice paper over the fillings, then fold the two sides flaps over the middle. Finally, roll the packet toward the back edge of the rice paper, creating a tight spring roll. The damp rice paper will stick to itself.
• Set aside on a serving plate and continue with the remaining ingredients. Keep the serving plate covered with a clean, damp towel until all spring rolls are prepared. Slice each roll once on the diagonal with a sharp knife and serve immediately with Peanut Butter Dipping Sauce.

Servings: 8

Nutrition Facts

Nutrition (per serving): 274 calories, 1.3g total fat, 412mg sodium, 43.8g carbohydrates, 1.4g fiber, 20.3g protein.

Roasted Red Pepper Dip

Colorful and delicious, this makes a large batch. If serving a smaller crowd, you may wish to cut the recipe in half.

1 cup roasted red peppers, jarred or home-roasted
1 tablespoon garlic-infused extra virgin olive oil
1 pound lactose-free cottage cheese
1 tablespoon fresh lemon juice
⅛ teaspoon white pepper
⅛ teaspoon Tabasco sauce (optional)

• Place all ingredients in a food processor bowl or blender. Process or blend until smooth and creamy.
• Serve chilled, with tortilla chips or fresh vegetables.

Servings: 16

Nutrition Facts

Nutrition (per serving): 30 calories, 1.1g total fat, 115mg sodium, 1.3g carbohydrates, <1g fiber, 3.6g protein.

Spinach Quesadillas

This is a low-FODMAP version of a perennial favorite. Corn tortillas aren't anything special right out of the bag, but warm them up in a skillet and they are downright delicious.

2 teaspoons olive oil
4 (6-inch) corn tortillas
1 cup mozzarella cheese, shredded
1 cup baby spinach leaves
½ cup roasted red peppers, chopped

- Drizzle olive oil into a cold skillet or onto an electric griddle. Turn the heat up to a medium-high setting. Place the corn tortillas on the griddle. Sprinkle first with grated cheese, then with spinach leaves and chopped roasted red peppers. When cheese has melted and spinach leaves are wilted, fold each quesadilla in half.
- Remove to a cutting board and cut in wedges. Serve warm.

Servings: 8

Nutrition Facts

Nutrition (per serving): 84 calories, 4.3g total fat, 79mg sodium, 7.1g carbohydrates, <1g fiber, 4.6g protein.

Warm Spinach Dip

This dip is warm and bubbly. It tastes great with corn chip or rice crackers.

2 teaspoons garlic-infused extra virgin olive oil
½ cup mayonnaise
½ cup plus 2 tablespoons Parmesan cheese, grated
8 ounces Neufchatel cheese, softened
¼ teaspoon freshly-ground black pepper, freshly ground
2 (9-ounce) packages frozen chopped spinach, prepared and squeezed dry

- Preheat oven to 350° F. Spread a 9" by 9" baking dish or pie plate with garlic-infused oil to add garlic flavor as well as to grease the baking dish.
- Combine mayonnaise, ½ cup Parmesan, and the Neufchatel cheese in a medium mixing bowl. Gently stir in the spinach. Transfer the mixture to the prepared baking dish and top with remaining 2 tablespoons Parmesan cheese.
- Bake until browned and bubbly, approximately 30 minutes.

Servings: 10

Nutrition Facts

Nutrition (per serving): 149 calories, 12g total fat, 392mg sodium, 5.8g carbohydrates, 1.6g fiber, 6.1g protein.

Dressings, Sauces, and Condiments

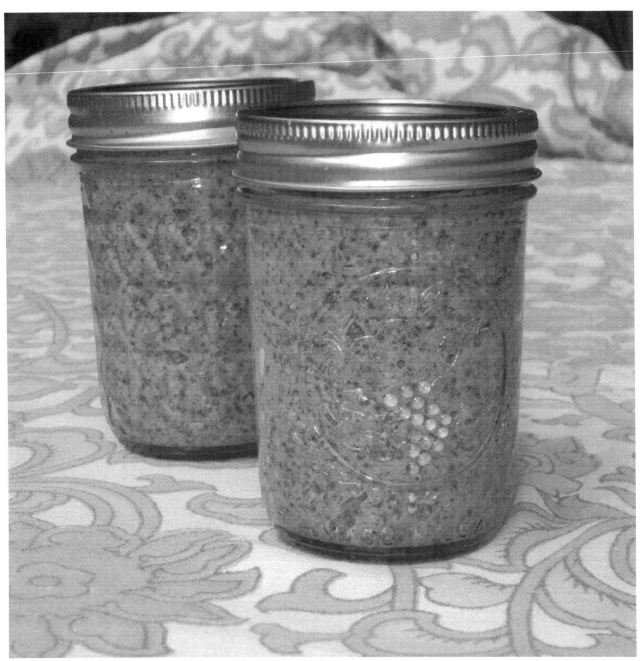

Brown Maple Mustard

Brown Maple Mustard

Timing is everything when making mustard, so observe the recommended time for each step of the process carefully for the best-tasting result.

½ cup yellow or white mustard seeds
½ cup brown or black mustard seeds
⅔ cup cold beer
¼ cup filtered cider vinegar
2 tablespoons 100% pure maple syrup
2 teaspoons salt

- Grind the yellow mustard seeds in a spice grinder or blender into a fine powder. Transfer the mustard flour to a small glass or ceramic mixing bowl.
- Grind the brown mustard seeds very briefly. Seeds should be just barely cracked to allow the liquid to soak in. Transfer the brown mustard seeds to the mixing bowl. Stir in the cold beer and allow the flour and seeds to soak for 10 minutes. Add the vinegar, maple syrup, and salt; stir to combine.
- Pour into a glass jar and store in the refrigerator for at least 2 days until serving.

Servings: 32, 1 tablespoon each

Nutrition Facts

Nutrition (per serving): 32 calories, 1.6g total fat, 146mg sodium, 3g carbohydrates, <1g fiber, 1.2g protein.

Recipe Tips

This mustard has quite a kick to it. You can turn down the heat by using more yellow mustard seeds and less brown ones. You can also use various liquids (water, wine, beer), various vinegars, and add horseradish or herbs.

Don't be alarmed if your mustard tastes terrible when it is freshly made. It must age at least 2 days for the bitterness to fade.

Spaghetti Sauce

Everyone needs a good red sauce in his or her repertoire. This sauce is easily put together. Serve over rice, corn, or quinoa pasta, or as a sauce for chicken or fish.

2 tablespoons olive oil or garlic-infused oil
1 bunch scallions, green part only, thinly sliced
1 (28-ounce) can diced tomatoes, drained
1 tablespoon dried basil, crushed
1 tablespoon dried oregano
2 teaspoons granulated sugar

- Measure garlic-infused oil into a 4-quart saucepan. Add scallions and sauté over medium heat for several minutes. Add remaining ingredients and cover the pot. Bring to a boil over medium-high heat, then reduce heat and simmer for approximately 30 minutes.
- If desired, use a stick blender to partially puree the sauce before serving.

Servings: 4, ½ cup each
Yield: 2 cups

Nutrition Facts

Nutrition (per serving): 110 calories, 7.2g total fat, 285mg sodium, 12g carbohydrates, 3.1g fiber, 2g protein.

Recipe Tips

For this recipe choose unseasoned, canned, diced tomatoes with tomato juice. No tomato concentrate, paste, or puree..

Blue Cheese Dressing

You might never want bottled blue cheese dressing again after enjoying this easy version.

　　　⅓ cup Gorgonzola or blue cheese, crumbled
　　　⅓ cup mayonnaise
　　　⅓ cup sour cream
　　　1 teaspoon lemon juice
　　　¼ teaspoon black pepper, freshly ground

- Combine ingredients in a small glass or ceramic bowl. Chill until serving.

　　　Servings: 8, 2 tablespoons each

Nutrition Facts

Nutrition (per serving): 76 calories, 6.8g total fat, 139mg sodium, 3g carbohydrates, <1g fiber, 1.4g protein.

Cranberry Orange Relish

This relish absolutely belongs on the dinner table at Thanksgiving.

　　　2 cups raw cranberries
　　　1 small organic navel orange
　　　1 cup granulated sugar

- Rinse the cranberries and scrub the orange. Cut the orange into quarters, but don't peel it. Pulse or grind the fruits together in a food processor or blender, until uniform small chunks are formed. Mixture should be coarse like crushed pineapple, not smooth like applesauce. Stir in sugar.
- Transfer to a glass jar, cover, and chill for two days before serving.

　　　Servings: 12, ¼ cup each

Nutrition Facts

Nutrition (per serving): 80 calories, <1g total fat, <1mg sodium, 20.6g carbohydrates, 1.2g fiber, <1g protein.

Zippy Ketchup

This ketchup has no high-fructose corn syrup, no onions, no garlic, and lots of zippy ketchup flavor. Maybe ketchup is a vegetable after all. The ground chia seeds help thicken this sauce.

　　　1 (14.5-ounce) can fire-roasted, diced tomatoes with juice
　　　1 tablespoon garlic-infused oil
　　　1 small red or green chili pepper, seeded (optional)
　　　⅓ cup brown sugar
　　　⅓ cup apple cider vinegar
　　　¼ teaspoon smoked paprika
　　　Pinch of ground allspice
　　　Pinch of ground cloves
　　　½ teaspoon salt
　　　1 tablespoon freeze dried chives or 2 tablespoons fresh snipped chives
　　　1 tablespoon ground chia seeds

- Combine all ingredients in a 3-quart saucepan. Bring the mixture to a boil over medium-high heat, reduce heat to low, and simmer for approximately 1 hour. Remove the ketchup from the heat and allow it to cool.
- Transfer the ketchup to a blender and puree. If the blender hasn't adequately pulverized the tomato seeds and skin, you can put the ketchup through a fine mesh strainer.
- Store the ketchup in a glass jar, tightly covered, in the refrigerator for up to two weeks.

Servings: 16, 2 tablespoons each

Nutrition Facts

Nutrition (per serving): 34 calories, 1.1g total fat, 111mg sodium, 6g carbohydrates, <1g fiber, <1g protein.

Recipe Tips

If you would like to add extra spices, such as cardamom or star anise, you may do so.
Works well as a barbecue sauce, too.

Jerk Marinade

This is a zingy marinade for whatever is going on the grill. Adapted from a recipe from Laura Molgaard.

¼ cup chives, snipped
1 red chili pepper , minced (optional)
juice of two limes
3 tablespoons olive oil
2 tablespoons tamari
1 tablespoon sugar
2 teaspoons black pepper
¾ teaspoon nutmeg, freshly grated
½ teaspoon ground cinnamon

- Puree all ingredients in a blender.
- Store in a covered jar in the refrigerator for up to 2 days before using to marinate chicken, pork, or fish for the grill. Discard marinade after use.

Servings: 6

Nutrition Facts

Nutrition (per serving): 82 calories, 6.9g total fat, 336mg sodium, 5.2g carbohydrates, <1g fiber, 1g protein.

Maple Mustard Dressing

Why pay several dollars a bottle for salad dressing when it is so easy to make a better one at home? This recipe has a hint of sweetness that pairs well with a spinach, slivered almond, and strawberry salad. Adapted from a recipe contributed by Nancy H.

¼ cup light olive oil
2 tablespoons filtered cider vinegar
2 tablespoons 100% pure maple syrup
2 teaspoons whole-grain mustard
¼ teaspoon paprika

- Combine all ingredients in a glass jar. Shake well. Chill until serving.

Servings: 8

Nutrition Facts

Nutrition (per serving): 75 calories, 6.9g total fat, 17mg sodium, 3.5g carbohydrates, <1g fiber, <1g protein.

Recipe Tips

Light olive oil is "light" in color and flavor compared to other olive oils; it is not low in calories. Other oils can be used in this recipe .
This recipe was tested with Grey Poupon Country Style Dijon mustard.

Lemon Curd

Delicious on crackers or muffins. The lemon zest adds intense flavor and interesting texture to the otherwise silky lemon curd.

10 tablespoons granulated sugar (½ cup plus 2 tablespoons)
2 large eggs
zest of two lemons (optional)
⅔ cup lemon juice, freshly squeezed (2-3 lemons)
3 tablespoons butter

- Combine all ingredients in a microwave safe bowl and whisk until smooth. Cook on high in the microwave for 30 seconds. Stir. Repeat. Lemon curd is done when it is thick enough to coat the back of a spoon.
- Remove from the microwave and pour into a glass jar. Cover. Store in the refrigerator and use within 1 week.

Servings: 16

Nutrition Facts

Nutrition (per serving): 61 calories, 2.8g total fat, 9mg sodium, 8.9g carbohydrates, <1g fiber, <1g protein.

Recipe Tips

Lemon "zest" is the finely grated or chopped outer rind of the lemon—just the flavorful yellow part with none of the white underneath.

Peanut Butter Dipping Sauce

This is a lovely sauce for grilled chicken, chicken satay, or fresh spring rolls.

6 tablespoons creamy peanut butter
2 tablespoons low-sodium soy sauce
½ cup coconut milk or cream
1 tablespoon ginger root, peeled and minced
2 teaspoons granulated sugar
1 teaspoon sesame oil, dark or spicy

- Stir all ingredients together in a medium-sized bowl or blender.
- Refrigerate for storage, but allow to come to room temperature before serving.

Servings: 8

Nutrition Facts

Nutrition (per serving): 111 calories, 9.7g total fat, 207mg sodium, 4.3g carbohydrates, <1g fiber, 3.6g protein.

Recipe Tips

Nutrient calculations reflect recipe prepared with coconut milk.
Water is a successful substitute for coconut milk in this recipe.

Salsa Ranchera

It will be hard to go back to ordinary salsa after sampling this flavorful, easy to assemble, party-sized version.

1 (28-ounce) can fire-roasted, diced tomatoes with juice
6 scallions, green part only, thinly-sliced
½ cup fresh cilantro, chopped
2 teaspoons garlic-infused extra virgin olive oil
½ teaspoon sea salt
juice of two limes

- Combine all ingredients in a glass or ceramic bowl. Cover and refrigerate for several hours to allow flavors to blend.
- May be served warm or cold.
  Servings: 6

Nutrition Facts

Nutrition (per serving): 45 calories, 1.7g total fat, 350mg sodium, 7.8g carbohydrates, 1.9g fiber, 1.5g protein.

Recipe Tips

This recipe was tested with Muir Glen Organic fire roasted diced tomatoes. Recipe can be halved easily, using a 14.5-ounce can of diced tomatoes.

Pineapple Salsa

Pineapple salsa pairs well with grilled or baked chicken, fish, or pork.

1 cup pineapple chunks, fresh, frozen, or canned
½ cup red bell pepper, seeded and cut into ¼-inch cubes
1 small red chili pepper , minced (optional)
¼ cup fresh cilantro, chopped
1 tablespoon fresh ginger, peeled and minced
juice of one lime

- Stir ingredients together or pulse gently in a blender or food processor.
- Store in a glass jar in the refrigerator for up to 2 days before serving.
  Servings: 4

Nutrition Facts

Nutrition (per serving): 50 calories, <1g total fat, 4mg sodium, 12.8g carbohydrates, 1.1g fiber, <1g protein.

Strawberry-Rhubarb Sauce

This sauce is delicious on pudding, ice cream, or toast.

½ cup granulated sugar
2 cups diced rhubarb
⅓ cup water
1 pound strawberries (2 ¾ cups), washed, hulled, and sliced
1 tablespoon lemon juice

- Combine sugar, rhubarb, and water in a heavy saucepan over medium-high heat. Bring to a boil, then reduce heat and simmer for 15 minutes. Add strawberries and lemon juice and simmer for 10 more minutes. Taste after 5 minutes and add a little more sugar if the mixture is too tart.
- Serve warm or cold. Store in a glass jar in the refrigerator for up to a week.
  Servings: 32, 2 tablespoons each

Nutrition Facts

Nutrition (per serving): 18 calories, <1g total fat, <1mg sodium, 4.6g carbohydrates, <1g fiber, <1g protein.

Turkey Gravy

A must-have for Thanksgiving dinner, this recipe works equally well with chicken broth for your Sunday chicken dinner.

**2 cups turkey or chicken broth from roasted bird
2 tablespoons cornstarch
4 tablespoons cold water
salt and black pepper, freshly ground, to taste**

- Place warm turkey or chicken broth in a medium saucepan.
- Combine cornstarch and cold water in a small bowl. Whisk the mixture into the broth. Stir the gravy over medium heat until it comes to a boil.
- Taste and season. Serve warm.

Servings: 8

Nutrition Facts

Nutrition (per serving): 74 calories, 7.4g total fat, 41mg sodium, 1.8g carbohydrates, <1g fiber, <1g protein.

Recipe Tips

If your roasted chick or turkey does not yield enough broth, add water to stretch it up to 2 cups or reduce the other ingredients proportionally to make a smaller batch.

Golden Syrup

Lyle's golden syrup appears frequently as an ingredient in recipes but can be difficult to find and very expensive in some parts of the world. Now you can make your own. Prepare this golden syrup the day before you plan to use it; you won't know if it turned out right until it has completely cooled.

**3 cups granulated cane sugar, divided
1 ¼ cups boiling water
2 lemon slices ¼-inch thick, with peel**

- Boil the water in a tea kettle or saucepan.
- Measure ½ cup sugar into a 3-quart heavy saucepan. Warm the sugar over medium heat, stirring constantly, until the sugar melts and turns into golden brown caramel. Remove from the heat, add the boiling water, and stir until all the caramel is dissolved. This may take 5 or 10 minutes.
- Add the remaining sugar and the lemon slices. Stir continuously while bringing the mixture to a boil over medium heat. Turn heat down to medium-low and simmer the uncovered syrup for 50 minutes. Do not stir again.
- Remove from heat and cool to room temperature. Check the consistency of the syrup. It should be much thicker than honey. It should slowly pour off a spoon in wide, thick ribbons. If the syrup is not thick enough, return it to the stove top and simmer for 10 more minutes. If it is too solid, gently re-warm it, add 2 tablespoons water, stir thoroughly until water is fully incorporated, and cool.
- Store, covered, in the refrigerator until use.

Servings: 20, 1 ½ tablespoons each
Yield: 2 ¼ cups

Nutrition Facts

Nutrition (per serving): 116 calories, 0g total fat, <1mg sodium, 30g carbohydrates, 0g fiber, 0g protein.

Bouquet Garni

These classic bundles of herbs add FODMAP-free flavor to your soups and stews, and lend a wonderful aroma to your kitchen.

3 sprigs fresh parsley
2 sprigs fresh thyme
1 fresh bay leaf

- Tie the bundle of herbs together with a piece of kitchen string.
- Use immediately to flavor any broth, soup, or stew by placing the bundle in the liquid during cooking. Remove the bundle of herbs before serving.

Tips

Bundles of bouquet garni can be dried for later use using a food dehydrator. If your oven can be set low enough, place bundled herbs on a wire cooling rack in the oven and bake for an hour at 125°F or until crisp. Store in a small airtight container.

When fresh herbs aren't available, combine 1 tablespoon of dried parsley, ½ tablespoon of dried thyme ,and a dried bay leaf. Place the mixture in a tea infuser or tie it up in a bundle of cheesecloth and remove before serving. Or put the herbs directly in the recipe and remove the bay leaf before serving. Experiment with sprigs of various additional herbs including rosemary and sage, if available.

Taco Seasoning Mix

This versatile seasoning works well in taco meat, sautéed tempe or tofu, Mexican-style rice, or rubbed on grilled steak or chicken.

2 tablespoons cornstarch
2 tablespoons ground chile powder
1 tablespoon ground cumin
½ teaspoon smoked paprika
1 teaspoon salt

- Combine dry ingredients and store in an airtight container.

Servings: 16, 1 teaspoon each
Yield: 16 teaspoons

Nutrition Facts

Nutrition (per serving): 8 calories, <1g total fat, 155mg sodium, 1.6g carbohydrates, <1g fiber, <1g protein.

Recipe Tips

Shop carefully for your ground chile peppers, which should be 100% chiles. "Chili powder" often has onion or garlic powder as part of the blend. 2 tablespoons of this mixture are enough to season 1 ½ pounds of ground beef or turkey, or 1 pound of sautéed tofu. Add ¼ cup water if desired.

Chocolate Syrup

This chocolate syrup is delicious served over ice cream, stirred into yogurt, or as an ingredient in smoothies and shakes.

> **1 cup water**
> **1 cup granulated sugar**
> **⅔ cup cocoa powder**
> **1 dash salt**
> **½ teaspoon vanilla extract**

- Combine water, sugar, cocoa powder, and salt in a medium saucepan. Stir constantly over medium heat until the mixture begins to simmer.
- Remove from heat and stir in vanilla.
- Transfer to a glass jar and refrigerate until serving.

> Servings: 16, 2 tablespoons each

Nutrition Facts

Nutrition (per serving): 57 calories, <1g total fat, 19mg sodium, 14.5g carbohydrates, 1.2g fiber, <1g protein.

Garlic-Infused Oil

This is a delicious way to get the flavor of garlic without the stomach ache, though it is less intense than commercial garlic oils. Use this as a cooking or flavoring oil to modify any recipe in your collection that calls for garlic.

> **½ cup extra-virgin olive oil**
> **3 large cloves garlic, washed, peeled, and crushed but still intact.**

- Pour olive oil into a small, heavy saucepan. Add large chunks of garlic. Heat oil until small bubbles rise vigorously from the garlic.
- Remove saucepan from the heat. The garlic will continue to cook. Allow garlic and oil to cool for a few minutes. Pour garlic and oil into a freshly washed glass jar with a cap or lid.
- Store in the refrigerator for up to a week.

> Servings: 8, 1 tablespoon each

Nutrition Facts

Nutrition (per serving): 121 calories, 13.5g total fat, <1mg sodium, <1g carbohydrates, <1g fiber, <1g protein.

Main Dishes

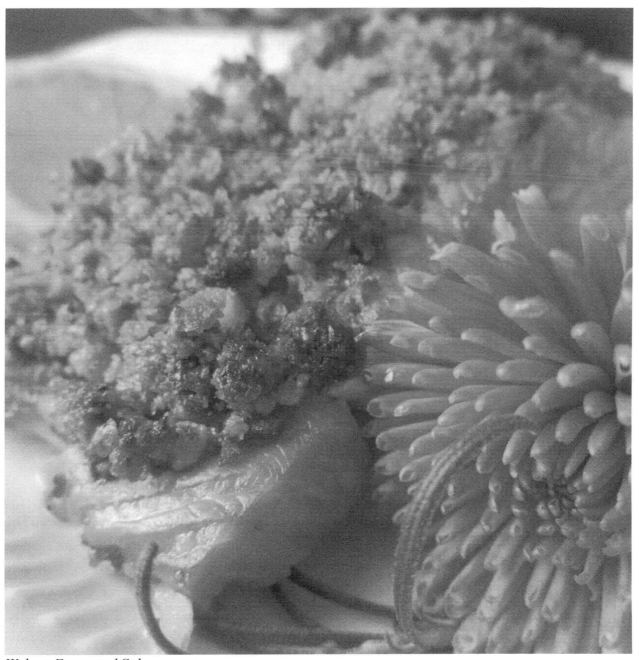

Walnut-Encrusted Salmon

Walnut-Encrusted Salmon

This very special dish can be started earlier in the day, then baked at the last minute. I guarantee your dinner guests will be impressed and their taste buds will be delighted.

> **½ cup walnut pieces**
> **2 tablespoons potato chips, crushed**
> **2 tablespoons lemon zest, grated**
> **1 teaspoon dried dill, or 1 tablespoon fresh dill, chopped**
> **1 tablespoon olive oil**
> **1 pound salmon filet**
> **2 tablespoons country style Dijon mustard**

- Preheat oven to 350° F.
- Grind walnuts, potato chips, lemon zest, dill, and olive oil together in a food processor or blender until crumbly. Divide salmon into 4 pieces and place skin side down in baking dish, with at least an inch between each piece. Spread mustard over the salmon filets. Spoon the crumb mixture over the filets and pat the crumbs down gently with a fork to make a ½-inch thick layer. Salt and pepper, if desired.
- Bake at 350° F for approximately 15 minutes or until fish flakes apart easily with a fork.
- Serve with lemon wedges, if desired.

> Servings: 4

Nutrition Facts

Nutrition (per serving): 382 calories, 27.7g total fat, 197mg sodium, 5.6g carbohydrates, 1.6g fiber, 28.4g protein.

Baked Meatballs

This recipe makes loads of meatballs, which can be frozen and added a few at a time to your favorite pasta or soup recipes.

> **2 pounds ground pork**
> **2 pounds 90% lean ground beef**
> **1 bunch fresh parsley, cleaned and chopped**
> **½ cup Parmesan cheese, grated**
> **2 large eggs, lightly beaten**
> **1 tablespoon Italian seasonings**
> **2 teaspoons salt**
> **1 teaspoon red pepper flakes (optional)**
> **½ cup quick cooking oats**

- Preheat oven to 400° F.
- Combine all ingredients in an extra large mixing bowl, using a sturdy wooden spoon or your hands. Form the meatballs into 30 2-inch balls with your hands or a small scoop and place on 2 large baking sheets. Baking sheets or pans must have edges to contain the juices that will be created during baking.
- Bake for approximately 50 minutes or until meatballs are browned and no pink remains in the center. Remove from the oven and drain hot fat off the cookie trays into a heat-proof, disposable container.
- Eat immediately or allow to cool before freezing in an airtight container.

> Servings: 30
> Yield: 30 large meatballs

Nutrition Facts

Nutrition (per serving): 158 calories, 10.5g total fat, 226mg sodium, 2.4g carbohydrates, <1g fiber, 12.9g protein.

Barbecued Brisket

This versatile recipe works equally well as the centerpiece of a holiday meal or a tailgate party. It is sized for a 2-quart slow cooker. If yours is larger, buy a bigger brisket and double the recipe.

> **2 pounds brisket or blade pot roast**
> **1 large clove garlic, halved**
> **½ cup beer**
> **2 tablespoons filtered cider vinegar**
> **1 tablespoon chili powder**
> **2 teaspoons sweet, smoked paprika**
> **¼ teaspoon ground cinnamon**
> **½ teaspoon kosher salt**
> **2 tablespoons light brown sugar, packed**
> **1 large fresh tomato, diced**

- Rub the inside of the slow cooker bowl with the cut sides of the garlic clove, then place the meat in the bowl, fatty side up.
- Combine the beer, vinegar, and all of the spices in a small bowl. Pour the mixture over the brisket. Add the chopped tomatoes. Cover the slow cooker and cook on low for 8-9 hours. Do not open the lid until at least 8 hours have passed. The meat should be tender, easily pierced and pulled apart with a fork.
- Remove the brisket to a serving platter and slice it. Pour a cup of the broth over the sliced brisket and serve.

Servings: 6

Nutrition Facts

Nutrition (per serving): 287 calories, 8.6g total fat, 242mg sodium, 7.8g carbohydrates, 1.1g fiber, 41.3g protein.

Risotto with Butternut Squash

This recipe does take some time at the stove, but the procedure is not difficult at all.

> **1 large clove garlic, slightly crushed but still intact**
> **2 tablespoons olive oil or garlic-infused oil**
> **1 cup Arborio rice, dry (no substitutions)**
> **3 cups Chicken Stock (recipe)**
> **1 cup white wine**
> **2 cups butternut squash, cooked and diced**
> **½ teaspoon red pepper flakes**
> **⅓ cup fresh Parmesan cheese, grated**
> **½ cup pumpkin seeds**

- Sauté rice and garlic in olive oil over medium heat in a large pot until well browned. Remove garlic.
- Combine the hot broth and white wine. Add the broth mixture ½ cup at a time, and stir every minute or 2 until it has been absorbed. Repeat. Continue until all the broth is used up and the rice is tender and creamy. Stir in remaining ingredients and allow to heat through. Season with salt and pepper if desired.
- Serve warm with extra cheese available at the table.

Servings: 4

Nutrition Facts

Nutrition (per serving): 572 calories, 22.3g total fat, 724mg sodium, 65.2g carbohydrates, 1.1g fiber, 21.5g protein.

Recipe Tips

The large pot seems like overkill for one cup of rice, but the large surface area on the bottom of the pot helps the risotto cook faster.

Braised Pork Chops with Orange Sauce

These pork chops are simple to prepare and have a complex flavor profile. The secret to this recipe is a heavy skillet with a tight-fitting lid.

6 boneless pork chops, about ¾-inch thick
⅛ teaspoon salt
⅛ teaspoon pepper
2 cloves garlic, peeled and quartered
1 tablespoon olive oil
2 teaspoons ginger root, peeled and minced
⅓ cup orange juice
3 tablespoons low-sodium soy sauce
1 tablespoon whole-grain mustard

- Place pork chops in a sealed zipper-top bag with the salt, pepper, olive oil and garlic. Manipulate the bag to mix the ingredients and coat the pork on all sides. Marinate in the refrigerator for at least 1 hour, or up to 24 hours.
- In a small bowl, combine the ginger, orange juice, soy sauce, and mustard. Set aside.
- Remove pork chops from bag and discard bag and garlic.
- Heat a large heavy skillet over medium-high heat. Brown the chops for 2 minutes per side. Pour the orange juice mixture over the chops. Move most of the ginger off the top of the chops so it can simmer in the sauce. Reduce heat to low, cover, and simmer for approximately 10-15 minutes or until pork is uniformly cooked.
- Serve chops together with warm sauce.

    Servings: 6

Nutrition Facts

Nutrition (per serving): 193 calories, 9.6g total fat, 431mg sodium, 2.9g carbohydrates, <1g fiber, 22.8g protein.

Crispy Baked Pork Chops

The low-FODMAP answer to Shake-n-Bake.

1 tablespoon olive oil
4 boneless pork chops, about ¾-inch thick
½ cup corn flakes, crushed

- Preheat oven to 400° F.
- Blot the pork chops dry with a paper towel (so the oil will stick). Drizzle the olive oil in a glass baking dish. Place the pork chops in the baking dish, moistening one side with oil. Turn the pork chops over and moisten the other side.
- Sprinkle the corn flake crumbs on a plate. One at a time, dredge the pork chops in the corn flake crumbs and return them to the baking dish. Sprinkle the remaining corn flake crumbs on top of the pork chops. Season with salt and pepper if desired.
- Bake 45 minutes.

    Servings: 4

Nutrition Facts

Nutrition (per serving): 249 calories, 10.5g total fat, 50mg sodium, 14.6g carbohydrates, <1g fiber, 22g protein.

Chef Salad

This salad goes together quickly when all the ingredients are on hand.

1 head romaine lettuce, torn in pieces
4 ounces cooked chicken or turkey, cut in strips
4 ounces ham, cut in strips
4 ounces Swiss cheese, cut in strips
2 large hard boiled eggs, sliced
1 large red bell pepper, seeded and chopped
2 medium tomatoes, cut in wedges
½ cup black olives

- Put romaine lettuce in a large salad bowl. Arrange remaining ingredients artistically on top of the lettuce.
- Serve with your choice of a FODMAP-friendly salad dressing or sprinkle with good quality olive oil and vinegar.

Servings: 5

Nutrition Facts

Nutrition (per serving): 218 calories, 11.5g total fat, 498mg sodium, 9.8g carbohydrates, 4.2g fiber, 20g protein.

Creamy Polenta with Zucchini

Polenta, Gorgonzola, and zucchini go together beautifully in this quick, weeknight supper.

4 ½ cups chicken stock or water, divided
1 cup cornmeal, coarsely ground
¼ teaspoon salt
⅔ cup Gorgonzola cheese, crumbled
1 tablespoon garlic-infused extra virgin olive oil
2 small Italian squash (zucchini), sliced ¼-inch thick
2 small summer squash, sliced ¼-inch thick
2 tablespoons cornstarch
½ cup fresh basil, chopped

- Bring 3 ½ cups of chicken broth to a boil in a medium saucepan. Slowly whisk in the cornmeal. Reduce heat to low and cook until very thick, about 10 minutes, stirring occasionally. Cooking time may vary depending on the type of cornmeal used. Stir in pepper and crumbled Gorgonzola. Remove from heat, cover, and set aside.
- Heat garlic-infused oil in a large non-stick skillet over medium-high heat until fragrant. Add zucchini and summer squash and cook, stirring occasionally for 10 minutes. Sprinkle the squash with cornstarch, and stir to coat. Add remaining cup of chicken broth and bring the mixture to a boil. Reduce heat to low and simmer for 2-3 minutes until sauce has thickened.
- Transfer the polenta to 4 bowls. Top with squash and sauce. Garnish with fresh basil and serve immediately.

Servings: 4

Nutrition Facts

Nutrition (per serving): 242 calories, 10.7g total fat, 437mg sodium, 31.9g carbohydrates, 3.7g fiber, 8.1g protein.

Recipe Tips

Recipe tested with Goya coarse yellow cornmeal.

Grilled Chicken Tidbits

Hats off to my sister-in-law Shelly for this one.

3 pounds boneless, skinless chicken thighs
1 teaspoon sea salt
1 tablespoon chili powder, or to taste
2 limes, juiced

- Slice chicken thighs in half length-wise on a large cutting board. Sprinkle with salt and chili powder on both sides and pack closely into a bowl or baking dish. Drizzle with the juice of 2 limes. Marinate for 6-8 hours.
- Cook on grill over medium heat, turning several times, until juices run clear and internal temperature of the chicken is 165° F.

Servings: 12

Nutrition Facts

Nutrition (per serving): 140 calories, 4.6g total fat, 260mg sodium, 1.5g carbohydrates, <1g fiber, 22.4g protein.

Curried Potato-Tuna Salad

This intriguing combination of ingredients will really surprise you. Try it, you'll like it.

1 ½ pounds Yukon Gold or other thin-skinned potatoes
2 tablespoons filtered cider vinegar
1 cup red or green grapes, halved
3 tablespoons mayonnaise
2 tablespoons plain lactose-free yogurt
2 tablespoons orange marmalade
1 ½ teaspoons Madras curry powder
½ teaspoon salt
½ teaspoon black pepper, freshly ground
1 (5-ounce) can tuna packed in water, drained
¼ cup sliced almonds, toasted
chives, snipped (optional)

- Scrub and cube the potatoes into bite-sized pieces, leaving the skins on. Cover with water in a medium saucepan and bring to a boil. Turn down heat and simmer until tender, approximately 20 minutes. Drain, sprinkle with cider vinegar, and set aside to cool.
- Combine mayo, yogurt, marmalade, curry powder, salt, and pepper in a large bowl and stir until smooth. Add the cooled or still slightly warm potatoes, and toss to coat.
- Just before serving, stir in toasted almonds and garnish with snipped chives if desired. Serve immediately, while slightly warm, or refrigerate until serving.

Servings: 6

Nutrition Facts

Nutrition (per serving): 281 calories, 9.7g total fat, 358mg sodium, 38.9g carbohydrates, 3.8g fiber, 11.4g protein.

Grilled Pork Tenderloin with Pancetta

This savory and decadent pork tenderloin is a real treat for meat lovers.

20 ounces pork tenderloin
1.5 ounces pancetta or prosciutto, thinly sliced
1 teaspoon black pepper, freshly ground

- Preheat the gas grill or burn charcoal briquettes until ashen on the outside, with cherry-red glow on the inside.
- Sprinkle the tenderloin with freshly ground black pepper. Wrap the tenderloin with overlapping thin slices of pancetta or prosciutto and secure with wooden skewers or cooking twine.
- Grill over a low-medium flame.
- When the pancetta is browned and crisp and a meat thermometer inserted into the center of the tenderloin reads 145° F, remove tenderloin to a serving platter, cover loosely with foil, and let it rest for 3 minutes. Carve into thin slices and serve warm

Servings: 5

Nutrition Facts

Nutrition (per serving): 301 calories, 13.1g total fat, 276mg sodium, 4.7g carbohydrates, <1g fiber, 37.3g protein.

Recipe Tips

Be sure to purchase an unprocessed cut of pork for this recipe, not a seasoned or marinated pork tenderloin.
Roasting in a 450° F oven for about 20 minutes or until the internal temperature reaches 145° F is another option for this recipe if no grill is available.

Macaroni and Cheese

Classic comfort food, straight from mom's oven.

8 ounces uncooked macaroni (rice, corn, or corn/quinoa)
2 tablespoons cornstarch
½ teaspoon salt
½ teaspoon dry mustard
¼ teaspoon black pepper, freshly ground
1 ¾ cups lactose-free milk
½ teaspoon red pepper flakes
2 cups Cheddar cheese, grated
1 ½ ounces potato chips, crumbled

- Preheat oven to 350° F. Grease a 9" by 9" baking dish with a few drops of oil or butter.
- Cook pasta according to package directions in an 8-quart saucepan. Do not overcook. Drain and set aside.
- Combine cornstarch, salt, dry mustard, and black pepper in the same saucepan. Add milk. Stir briskly until smooth. Bring to a boil over medium heat, stirring constantly with a wide, flat-edged, heat-safe spatula moving along the bottom of the saucepan. Remove from heat and stir in grated cheese and red pepper flakes. Add pasta, stir. Transfer the mixture to the greased baking dish. Sprinkle the potato chips on top of the casserole.
- Bake, uncovered, for 25 minutes or until lightly browned.

Servings: 4

Nutrition Facts

Nutrition (per serving): 542 calories, 24g total fat, 744mg sodium, 60.3g carbohydrates, 6.8g fiber, 22.7g protein.

Sizzling Beef Stir-Fry

For a delicious change of pace, try this stir-fried meal.

> 1 pound lean beef, very thinly sliced against the grain
> 1 teaspoon sesame oil
> 4 teaspoons garlic-infused extra virgin olive oil, divided
> 1 jalapeno pepper, seeded and minced (optional)
> 1 tablespoon fresh ginger, peeled and minced
> 2 tablespoons cornstarch
> 1 cup bean sprouts
> 3 ounces baby spinach leaves
> 1 small summer squash, sliced ¼-inch thick
> 1 tablespoon brown sugar
> 3 tablespoons reduced-sodium soy sauce
> 2 tablespoons sesame seeds, toasted

- Marinate the beef strips in the sesame oil, 1 teaspoon of the infused garlic oil, fresh ginger, and jalapenos for at least 1 hour in a glass bowl.
- Sprinkle the beef with cornstarch and stir to coat. Heat 1 tablespoon of garlic-infused oil in an extra large heavy skillet until fragrant and very hot. Add the steak and stir-fry for 3-4 minutes to brown the beef on all sides. Remove from the pan and set aside.
- Add the bean sprouts, spinach leaves, and summer squash to the skillet. Cook, stirring, until the spinach is wilted and summer squash is tender. Return the beef to the skillet. Add the soy sauce and brown sugar and stir for another minute.
- Remove from heat, sprinkle with sesame seeds, and serve over rice or rice noodles.

> Servings: 4

Nutrition Facts

Nutrition (per serving): 290 calories, 14.4g total fat, 618mg sodium, 12.6g carbohydrates, 1.8g fiber, 27.7g protein

Salmon Platter

Serve this dish for your cocktail party or buffet dinner. This must be made ahead—no last minute fussing.

> 2 pounds salmon filet
> 1 bunch fresh dill
> 2 medium fresh lemons, sliced into thin rounds
> ½ cup plain lactose-free yogurt
> 1 teaspoon garlic-infused extra virgin olive oil
> ½ cup mayonnaise
> ¼ teaspoon salt
> ¼ teaspoon black pepper, freshly ground

- Place salmon filet skin side down on a baking sheet. Bake at 400° F approximately 10 minutes per inch of thickness. Check to see if the fish is done by using two forks to gently pull apart the flesh at the thickest part of the filet. If it pulls apart easily and is uniformly opaque inside, it is done. Remove fish from oven and carefully scrape off any congealed protein on top of the filet. Allow the fish to cool until it can be handled safely.
- Using 2 spatulas, transfer the entire filet to a large platter; it's OK if the skin stays behind on the baking sheet.
- Finely chop the dill, reserving a few heads for garnish. Combining chopped dill, yogurt, mayonnaise, garlic-infused oil, salt and black pepper to taste.

- Arrange the lemon slices and dill heads on the cooled fish in a pleasing way. Put a small bowl of the sauce either on or beside the serving platter.

Servings: 10

Nutrition Facts

Nutrition (per serving): 286 calories, 21.2g total fat, 181mg sodium, 3.3g carbohydrates, 1.1g fiber, 21g protein.

Quinoa Veggie Burgers

These burgers are delicious hot or cold, so make extras for the lunch box.

½ cup dry, pre-rinsed quinoa
1 ½ cups water
2 tablespoons garlic-infused oil or olive oil
¾ cup carrots, diced
¼ cup scallions, green part only, thinly sliced
¼ cup red bell pepper, seeded and diced
¼ cup frozen green peas, thawed
¼ teaspoon salt
pinch of cayenne pepper
1 tablespoon fresh thyme leaves (or 1 teaspoon dried)
2 teaspoons fresh rosemary, minced (or ½ teaspoon dried)
2 tablespoons brown rice flour
¼ cup fresh flat-leaf parsley, minced
½ cup old-fashioned oats
2 egg whites, slightly beaten

- Toast quinoa in 3- or 4-quart sauce pan until fragrant (about 3 minutes). Add water and bring to a boil. Reduce heat and simmer until the water is absorbed, approximately 15 minutes. Remove from heat and set aside.
- Heat 2 tablespoons of garlic-infused oil in a medium sauté pan over medium heat. Add carrots and green onions. Cook for 3 minutes. Add red bell pepper, salt, cayenne, thyme, and rosemary. Cook for 3 more minutes, stirring occasionally. Reduce heat to medium-low and continue to cook until vegetables are tender and moisture is evaporated, approximately 5-7 minutes. Add green peas and remove from heat. Combine quinoa and sautéed vegetables and allow the mixture to cool for approximately 20 minutes.
- Preheat oven to 350° F.
- Sprinkle mixture with brown rice flour and gently stir to combine. Add parsley, oats, and beaten egg whites. Mold mixture into 5 large patties and set on a parchment lined baking sheet. Place in the freezer for 20 minutes or in the fridge for 1 hour to set.
- Bake in oven for 25 minutes, flipping patties half way through cook time.

Servings: 5

Nutrition Facts

Nutrition (per serving): 210 calories, 7.8g total fat, 169mg sodium, 28.2g carbohydrates, 4.4g fiber, 7.6g protein.

Lemon Sole

Delicately flavored, quick, and easy, this recipe is ready to serve in 10 minutes.

> 1 ¼ pounds filet of sole, flounder, or other white fish
> ⅓ cup rice flour
> ½ teaspoon salt
> ½ teaspoon black pepper, freshly ground
> 1 tablespoon butter
> 1 tablespoon olive oil
> 4 tablespoons almonds, sliced and toasted
> 2 tablespoons coarsely chopped fresh parsley
> 1 lemon, cut into wedges

- Place fish filets into a gallon plastic zipper bag with ½ cup rice flour, salt, and pepper. Close the bag securely and shake it until filets are evenly coated with flour. Add a little more rice flour if needed.
- Melt the butter and oil in a large heavy skillet over medium-high heat. Cook the filets for 2-3 minutes on each side until golden brown. Fish is done when it flakes easily and flesh is opaque all the way through. Remove to plates.
- Garnish fish with toasted almonds, chopped parsley, and lemon wedges.

> Servings: 4

Nutrition Facts

Nutrition (per serving): 289 calories, 12.9g total fat, 408mg sodium, 13.3g carbohydrates, 1.8g fiber, 29.7g protein.

Recipe Tips

Trader Joe's toasted sliced almonds can't be beat.

Mediterranean Shrimp Salad

This dish is a real treat, and can easily handle variations in the type and amount of rice, protein, and vegetables.

> 2 cups brown rice, cooked
> 9 ounces shrimp, peeled, cooked, and deveined
> 1 cup cucumber peeled, seeded, and cut into ¼-inch cubes
> 3 tablespoons chopped fresh basil
> 3 tablespoons chopped parsley
> ½ cup red bell pepper, seeded and cut into ¼-inch cubes
> 1 cup frozen green peas, thawed
> ½ cup feta cheese, crumbled
> ¼ teaspoon salt
> ¼ teaspoon black pepper
> 2 tablespoons extra virgin olive oil
> 2 tablespoons red wine vinegar

- Thaw shrimp and green peas, if frozen.
- Combine ingredients in large bowl. Chill until serving.

> Servings: 4

Nutrition Facts

Nutrition (per serving): 320 calories, 12.5g total fat, 542mg sodium, 30.4g carbohydrates, 3.9g fiber, 20.6g protein.

Mom's Meatloaf

Roasted red peppers add both color and flavor to this variation on a traditional meatloaf.

1 (12-ounce) jar roasted red peppers, divided
1 pound ground pork
1 ½ pounds lean ground beef
2 large eggs, lightly beaten
½ cups quick oats
½ teaspoon salt
1 teaspoon Italian seasoning
½ teaspoon red pepper flakes (optional)

- Preheat oven to 375° F.
- Drain the roasted red peppers. Chop half of them and purée the rest. Set both aside.
- Combine ground pork and beef in a large mixing bowl. Stir in the chopped red pepper, beaten egg, oatmeal, salt, dried herbs, and red pepper flakes using a large fork. Transfer the meat mixture to an 8" by 8" glass baking dish or two 9" by 5" glass loaf pans.
- Bake for 30 minutes.
- Remove from the oven, and spread the red pepper purée over the top of the meatloaf. Return to the oven and bake for 30 more minutes. Drain the fat from the around the edges of the meatloaf and serve hot.

    Servings: 9

Nutrition Facts

Nutrition (per serving): 370 calories, 27.7g total fat, 225mg sodium, 4.3g carbohydrates, <1g fiber, 24g protein.

Recipe Tips

Bake 1 loaf pan today; cover the other with plastic wrap, then aluminum foil, and freeze for another day.

Near East Chicken Salad

A main dish salad with the exotic flavors of the East, this is an outstanding light meal or buffet dish. If you can't eat sour cream, double up on the mayo.

½ cup mayonnaise
½ cup sour cream
¼ cup marmalade
3 tablespoons lemon juice, freshly squeezed
1 ½ teaspoons Madras curry powder
½ teaspoon cumin
½ teaspoon coriander
¼ teaspoon black pepper, freshly ground
½ cup red bell pepper, chopped
2 ½ cups brown Basmati rice, freshly cooked
2 cups seedless grapes, halved
2 cups cooked chicken or turkey, cubed

- Combine mayonnaise, sour cream, marmalade, lemon juice, and spices in a large bowl. Add remaining ingredients and stir gently to evenly distribute the dressing.
- Serve on spring greens and sprinkle with slivered almonds, if desired.

    Servings: 6

Nutrition Facts

Nutrition (per serving): 359 calories, 13.2g total fat, 197mg sodium, 43.7g carbohydrates, 2.5g fiber, 18g protein.

Rice Noodle Bowl for One

Dining alone? This noodle bowl can be assembled in just a few minutes using low-FODMAP pantry staples like rice noodles, frozen cooked shrimp, peanuts, and whatever vegetables you have on hand.

      3 large shrimp, peeled, cooked, deveined
      1 ½ ounces rice sticks
      2 teaspoons low-sodium soy sauce
      1 teaspoon sugar
      ½ teaspoon chili-flavored sesame oil
      ½ teaspoon garlic-infused oil
      1 tablespoon rice vinegar
      ½ cup red peppers, thinly sliced
      ½ cup cooked sweet potato, peeled and cubed
      ½ cup bok choy, thinly sliced
      1 tablespoon peanuts, crushed

- Place rice sticks in a large soup bowl and cover with boiling water. Let them soak for 5-7 minutes.
- Meanwhile, whisk together soy sauce, sugar, chili oil, and rice vinegar in a small bowl. Set aside.
- Heat garlic-infused oil in a small skillet over medium-high heat. Add vegetables and stir-fry for 1 minute. Add soy sauce mixture and cook for another minute.
- Drain rice sticks, and top with vegetables, sauce, and shrimp. Sprinkle with crushed peanuts.

     Servings: 1

Nutrition Facts

Nutrition (per serving): 219 calories, 9.1g total fat, 432mg sodium, 33.2g carbohydrates, 3.4g fiber, 8g protein.

Zucchini Frittata

This is nice for breakfast or for a quick weeknight supper.

      2 tablespoons extra virgin olive oil
      ¾ pound zucchini, thinly sliced
      6 large eggs, beaten
      ½ cup ricotta cheese
      1 tablespoon fresh herbs or ¼ teaspoon dried
      ⅓ cup Parmesan cheese, grated
      salt and black pepper, freshly ground, to taste

- Heat the olive oil in a 10″ or 12″ non-stick skillet over medium heat until fragrant. Sauté zucchini until tender and lightly browned, stirring frequently.
- Meanwhile, combine beaten eggs, lactose-free ricotta cheese, and your preferred fresh or dried herbs. Pour egg mixture over browned zucchini in the same skillet. As the frittata cooks, lift the edges and tilt the pan to allow egg mixture to run underneath. Continue cooking until the top is beginning to set. Use a large spatula to flip the entire frittata and cook the top side briefly.
- Sprinkle with grated Parmesan cheese, turn the heat off, and cover for 2-3 minutes, or until cheese is somewhat melted. Salt and pepper, if desired, and serve in wedges.

     Servings: 3

Nutrition Facts

Nutrition (per serving): 345 calories, 25.6g total fat, 372mg sodium, 7.2g carbohydrates, 1.3g fiber, 22.9g protein.

Pancetta-Spinach Frittata

This filling meal can be on the table in 30 minutes or less.

6 large eggs, slightly beaten
½ cup ricotta cheese
½ cup pancetta, diced
1 cup baby spinach leaves
½ teaspoon salt
¼ teaspoon pepper
¼ teaspoon sweet, smoked paprika
2 teaspoons olive oil
½ cup grape tomatoes, halved
½ cup Cheddar cheese, grated

- Preheat oven to 350° F.
- Whisk together eggs, ricotta, and pancetta. Add salt, pepper, and paprika and whisk to combine.
- Heat olive oil over medium-high heat in an 8" or 9" oven-proof skillet. Add baby spinach and pancetta and cook until wilted. Pour on egg mixture and cook until edge sets, about 4 minutes. Lift the edges with a spatula several times and allow uncooked egg mixture to run to the edge and under the frittata. Arrange grape tomato halves on top of the egg mixture. Sprinkle with grated cheese.
- Place skillet in the preheated oven and bake until the center of the frittata is slightly firm to the touch, approximately 15 minutes.
- Serve warm frittata in wedges.

Servings: 3

Nutrition Facts

Nutrition (per serving): 356 calories, 24.6g total fat, 1072mg sodium, 5.6g carbohydrates, <1g fiber, 28.4g protein.

Recipe Tips

If pancetta isn't available, diced ham or precooked chicken sausage will do nicely as a substitute.

If you don't have an oven-proof skillet, you can turn the stove top burner down to low, cover the skillet, and wait a few minutes for the cheese to melt.

Shrimp and Grits

I had my first marvelous taste of shrimp and grits recently during a visit to North Carolina. I love living in New England, but I'm feeling a bit robbed by all the years of shrimp and grits I've missed. This is my no onion, no garlic rendition of this southern classic.

1 cup grits, coarsely ground, dry, prepared according to package directions
1 tablespoon garlic-infused extra virgin olive oil
1 cup Cheddar cheese, grated
1 pound raw shrimp, peeled and deveined
4 slices thickly-cut bacon
Juice of half a lemon
2 tablespoons chopped parsley
1 bunch scallions, green part only, thinly sliced

- Bring the water and salt to a boil in a 4-quart saucepan with a heavy lid. Gradually whisk the grits into the boiling water. Cover the pot, turn the heat down to low, and simmer until the water is absorbed, approximately 30 minutes. Remove from heat and stir in garlic-infused oil and cheese. Cover and set aside.
- Fry the bacon in a large heavy skillet until crisp. Remove the bacon to drain on a paper towel, then chop and set aside. Pour off all but a thin layer of bacon grease. Add shrimp to the hot grease and cook briefly until shrimp begin to turn pink. Add the lemon juice, chopped bacon, parsley, and scallions and sauté for several minutes. Shrimp are done when they are opaque white throughout. Do not overcook.
- Divide grits into 4 serving bowls and top with the shrimp mixture. Sprinkle with some extra shredded Cheddar cheese, if desired. Serve immediately.

Servings: 4

Nutrition Facts

Nutrition (per serving): 588 calories, 32.3g total fat, 662mg sodium, 34g carbohydrates, <1g fiber, 38.1g protein.

Recipe Tips

Tested with Trader Joe stone ground grits. These grits are very coarsely ground; finely ground grits don't make a good substitute.

Tempeh Fried Rice

This recipe is a great way to use up leftovers, and any available protein food may be used in place of tempeh. When I cook rice for dinner I often make extra in anticipation of making this family favorite the following night.

2 tablespoons garlic-infused oil
2 large eggs, lightly beaten (optional)
4 tablespoons low-sodium soy sauce
2 ½ tablespoons peanut butter
1 tablespoon brown sugar, packed
1 tablespoon rice vinegar
1 tablespoon garlic-infused oil
2 teaspoons dark or spicy sesame oil
¼ teaspoon black pepper, freshly ground
1 cup carrots, peeled and shredded
4 cups rice, cooked and chilled
½ pound tempeh
1 cup bok choy, chopped
1 cup pineapple chunks, drained
½ cup peanuts
1 small bunch scallions, green part only, thinly sliced

- Heat ½ tablespoon garlic oil over medium-high heat in a large non-stick skillet. Add the eggs and cook, stirring constantly with a wooden or silicone spoon, until firm but not browned. Set aside.
- In a separate bowl, combine soy sauce, peanut butter, brown sugar, rice vinegar, garlic-infused oil, sesame oil, black pepper, and hot sauce. Set aside.
- Heat remaining garlic oil in the skillet until it spatters when a drop of water is dropped in the pan. Add carrots to the pan and sauté until tender. Transfer the chilled rice to the skillet and cook, stirring occasionally, for 5-10 minutes until rice is heated through and slightly crispy in parts. Add remaining ingredients and prepared sauce, and continue to cook, stirring occasionally until heated through.
- Serve immediately.
    Servings: 5

Nutrition Facts

Nutrition (per serving): 565 calories, 29.1g total fat, 623mg sodium, 59.7g carbohydrates, 3.9g fiber, 21.8g protein.

Warm Chicken and Rice Salad

This easy recipe takes the place of a turkey sandwich in your lunch box. It goes together quickly using the meat from a grocery store rotisserie chicken. It also makes a welcome contribution to a potluck supper.

2 cups Jasmine rice, dry
3 cups water
¼ cup pine nuts or walnuts
1 ½ cups frozen baby peas
3 cups cooked chicken, diced
1 ½ teaspoons lemon peel, grated (optional)
2 lemons, juiced
¼ cup extra virgin olive oil
1 (11-ounce) can mandarin oranges, drained
¼ cup minced parsley
1 teaspoon salt, or to taste
½ teaspoon pepper, freshly ground

- Rinse Jasmine rice to remove excess starch.
- Bring water to a boil in a medium saucepan, add the rice, reduce the heat and simmer for 25 minutes. Remove from heat and set aside.
- Meanwhile, in a small frying pan, toast the pine nuts over low heat, stirring frequently, for 3-5 minutes. Set aside.
- Rinse frozen baby peas to thaw slightly, but don't cook them. Grate or finely chop lemon zest from whole lemons before halving the lemons and squeezing out the juice. Combine all ingredients in an extra large bowl. Taste for seasonings, and adjust salt and pepper, if necessary.
- Serve warm or cold.
    Servings: 6

Nutrition Facts

Nutrition (per serving): 407 calories, 13.7g total fat, 450mg sodium, 59.6g carbohydrates, 2.9g fiber, 11.4g protein.

Recipe Tips

1 ½ pounds raw, boneless chicken will yield a little over 3 cups cooked chicken.

Vegetarian Shepherd's Pie

This vegetarian version of shepherd's pie uses protein-rich seitan in place of meat. Make the seitan a day ahead to break up the work load.

> ¼ cup garlic-infused extra virgin olive oil
> 1 recipe "Chicken" Seitan, approximately 1 ½ pounds, cubed
> ½ cup red wine
> 2 cups hot water
> 1 teaspoon Italian seasoning
> 1 pound peas and carrots, frozen
> ¼ cup melted butter
> ¼ cup sorghum flour
> 2 ½ pounds potatoes, peeled and diced
> 1 cup lactose-free milk
> ½ cup Cheddar cheese, shredded

- Heat the olive oil in a 6- or 8-quart soup pot over medium-high heat. Add seitan and sauté until browned, turning occasionally, for 5-10 minutes. Add wine, water, and Italian seasoning. Bring to a boil and simmer for 20 minutes. Add carrots and peas and simmer for 10 more minutes.
- Meanwhile, cover potatoes with cold water in a 4-quart saucepan. Bring to a boil, then reduce heat and simmer potatoes until tender, approximately 15 minutes. Drain and mash the potatoes, then add milk, Cheddar cheese, salt, and pepper. Set aside.
- Melt butter in a small bowl. Stir in sorghum flour to make a roux (paste of butter and flour). Drop the roux by spoonfuls into the simmering stew. Stir briskly to combine after each spoonful. When gravy has thickened, remove from heat.
- Preheat broiler, and grease a 9" by 13" baking dish with butter or oil. Transfer the stew into the baking dish. Spoon potato mixture over stew and spread evenly to cover. Broil about 3 inches from the top heating element in the oven until top is golden brown, about 10 minutes.

Servings: 8

Nutrition Facts

Nutrition (per serving): 418 calories, 16.1g total fat, 484mg sodium, 34.1g carbohydrates, 4.1g fiber, 34.1g protein.

Recipe Tips

Use lean ground beef or turkey for this recipe instead of seitan if you prefer; cook and drain the meat before proceeding with the recipe. Or, use tempeh for a gluten-free, vegan version.

Tempeh Nuggets

These flavorful protein nuggets can top a salad, a stir-fry, or a pizza. Tempeh is a fermented soybean product with a nutty flavor that is lower in FODMAPs than other legumes, according to researchers at Monash University. Processing varies, so check the ingredients to make sure no FODMAPs were added, and try a small portion of your brand at first, to make sure you tolerate it.

> 8 ounces tempeh
> 4 teaspoons garlic-infused oil, divided
> 3 tablespoons balsamic vinegar
> 1 tablespoon reduced-sodium soy sauce
> ¼ teaspoon red pepper flakes, or more to taste
> ¼ teaspoon dried thyme leaves, crushed
> 1 teaspoon dried basil
> 1 teaspoon dried rosemary, crushed

- Cut the tempeh into bite-sized pieces and place in a medium-sized bowl. Add 2 teaspoons of the garlic-infused oil along with the remaining ingredients and stir to coat. Cover the bowl and marinate in the refrigerator for at least 1 hour. Stir occasionally.
- Heat the remaining 2 teaspoons of garlic-infused oil in a large non-stick skillet over medium heat until it's fragrant. Transfer the tempeh and any remaining marinade to the skillet. Cook the tempeh, turning frequently until all liquid has evaporated and the nuggets begin to caramelize. Give this your full attention, as it scorches easily.
- Eat immediately or chill for use in other recipes as desired.

  Servings: 3

Nutrition Facts

Nutrition (per serving): 219 calories, 14.3g total fat, 211mg sodium, 11g carbohydrates, <1g fiber, 14.5g protein.

Recipe Tips

2 ½ teaspoons of Italian seasoning can be used in place of individual dried herbs. Herbs can be varied to suit your recipe.
The recipe was tested with Lightlife Organic soy tempeh. Read tempeh ingredients carefully. It often has other high-FODMAP ingredients added.

Pan Fried Tofu

Tofu is the low-FODMAP answer to getting enough protein on a vegetarian or vegan diet, and it is surprisingly easy to prepare. These crispy, pan-fried tofu nuggets can stand in for the meat, fish, or poultry in many of the recipes in this book, or can be served on their own.

1 pound extra- firm tofu
3 tablespoons cornstarch
¼ teaspoon salt
½ teaspoon herb or spice of your choice
1 tablespoon garlic-infused oil

- Slice tofu into ½-inch thick sheets. Place between layers of clean paper towels or dishcloths and weigh down with a heavy object for at least 30 minutes.
- Cut the tofu into uniformly sized bite-sized pieces and toss them in a bowl with the cornstarch, salt, and seasoning.
- Heat the olive oil in a large non-stick skillet over medium heat until fragrant. Add the tofu in a single layer. Don't crowd the tofu—this might mean frying it in two batches, with a little extra oil. Cook the tofu for 3-4 minutes on each side, until golden brown and crispy.
- Eat the tofu as is, or include it in recipes as desired.

  Servings: 4

Nutrition Facts

Nutrition (per serving): 499 calories, 10g total fat, 163mg sodium, 89.9g carbohydrates, 1.3g fiber, 11.5g protein.

Recipe Tips

Brown rice flour and/or sesame seeds are other options for coating the tofu before frying, if you don't wish to use cornstarch.
Possible seasonings: ground chiles, Italian seasoning, Bell's poultry seasoning, Tajin Clásico Seasoning.

"Chicken" Seitan

Seitan is a high-protein meat substitute made from wheat gluten. Use chicken seitan as a substitute in any of your favorite recipes. It's delicious grilled or as a pizza topping.

1 (10 ounce) box vital wheat gluten
1 tablespoon Bell's poultry seasoning
¼ teaspoon garlic-infused oil
⅓ cup low-sodium soy sauce or water
10 cups water, divided
¼ cup scallions, thinly sliced, green part only
⅛ teaspoon black pepper, freshly ground

- Mix vital wheat gluten, Bell's poultry seasoning, and garlic-infused olive oil in a large glass bowl. Stir until very uniform mixture is formed. Add soy sauce and 2 cups of water. Stir until gluten develops into a rubbery ball. Place the dough on a clean counter top. Knead it a few times and shape it into a log about the diameter of your fist. Set the dough aside for 15 minutes while making the stock.
- Bring 8 cups of water, scallions, and pepper to a boil in a large stockpot. Cut the gluten into desired shapes and drop the pieces into the boiling stock. Reduce heat to low, cover, and simmer for 45 minutes.
- Remove seitan from stock and cool on a plate. Refrigerate or freeze until using in your favorite recipes.

Servings: 12

Nutrition Facts

Nutrition (per serving): 93 calories, <1g total fat, 249mg sodium, 4.1g carbohydrates, <1g fiber, 18.1g protein.

Side Dishes

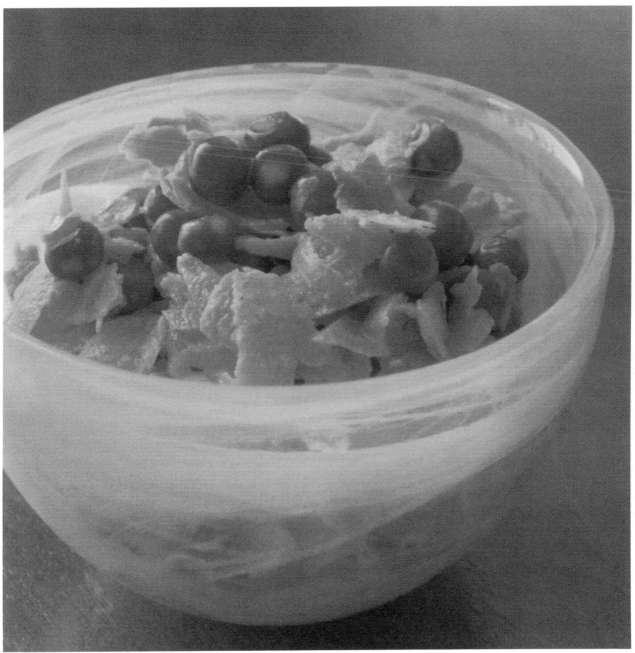

Lemony Carrot and Pea Salad

Lemony Carrot and Pea Salad

Make a double batch of this in place of coleslaw for your next backyard party.

   ½ pound carrots, peeled and shredded
   1 cup frozen green peas, thawed
   ⅓ cup mayonnaise
   1 small lemon, juiced
   ½ teaspoon granulated sugar
   ¼ teaspoon salt
   ⅛ teaspoon black pepper, freshly ground

- Combine mayonnaise, lemon juice, sugar, salt, and pepper in a medium bowl. Add carrots and peas; stir gently.
- Serve chilled.

   Servings: 6

Nutrition Facts

Nutrition (per serving): 88 calories, 4.5g total fat, 242mg sodium, 11.1g carbohydrates, 2.1g fiber, 1.8g protein.

Quinoa Pilaf

This is a versatile recipe that can accommodate whatever FODMAP-friendly vegetables you have on hand in place of those suggested.

   1 cup quinoa, dry
   2 cups water
   2 tablespoons olive oil
   1 cup sweet potato, cooked, peeled, and cubed
   ½ teaspoon salt
   ⅛ teaspoon black pepper, freshly ground
   1 cup cherry tomatoes, halved
   ¼ cup pecan pieces, toasted
   1 bunch scallions, green part only, thinly sliced
   ¼ cup fresh basil, chopped
   juice of a whole lime

- Measure quinoa into a medium sauce pan then add 2 cups water. Bring to a boil, then turn down heat and simmer until the water is absorbed, about 10-15 minutes. Remove from heat and allow to cool briefly. Add remaining ingredients and stir gently to combine.
- Serve warm as a side dish.

   Servings: 6

Nutrition Facts

Nutrition (per serving): 181 calories, 6.6g total fat, 214mg sodium, 26.3g carbohydrates, 3.8g fiber, 5.3g protein.

Recipe Tips

Vary the seasonings to suit yourself. Orange juice and grated ginger might be nice in place of the lime juice and fresh basil.
Unless you are certain the quinoa has been pre-rinsed, do it yourself. Rinsing removes the naturally occurring soap-like saponins from the quinoa, which will improve its taste. A large, fine-mesh strainer is the easiest way to rinse the grain.
Leftovers will make a delicious cold salad. Just add chunks of chicken or shrimp for lunch the next day.

Creamy Mashed Potatoes for Two

You can enjoy mashed potatoes even if you are lactose intolerant with the help of lactose-free milk.

2 medium potatoes
¼ cup lactose-free milk
1 tablespoon butter
2 tablespoons sour cream
⅛ teaspoon salt
⅛ teaspoon black pepper, freshly ground

- Scrub, peel, and rinse the potatoes. Slice them into ½-inch thick slices, place them in a 4-quart saucepan, and cover the potatoes with cool water. Bring the potatoes to a boil over high heat in the uncovered saucepan. Cover the pan, reduce the heat to low, and simmer until potatoes are tender, about 12-15 minutes. Drain the boiling water off, leaving potatoes in the warm saucepan. Add butter, lactose-free milk, salt, pepper, and optional seasonings (see tips). Mash the potatoes using a potato masher. Stir in low-fat sour cream.
- Serve warm.

Servings: 2

Nutrition Facts

Nutrition (per serving): 254 calories, 8.8g total fat, 218mg sodium, 39.3g carbohydrates, 4.7g fiber, 5.8g protein.

Recipe Tips

Optional seasonings, if available, could include fresh snipped herbs (chives, scallion greens, rosemary, or parsley) or 2 teaspoons of prepared horseradish.

Coconut Basmati Rice

People on low-FODMAP diets tend to eat a lot of rice. For a pleasant change, try this fragrant basmati rice with your next meal.

1 tablespoon butter
1 ½ cups brown basmati rice, dry
2 tablespoons coconut flakes, unsweetened
1 (14-ounce) can coconut milk
1 cup water
½ teaspoon salt
1 cardamom pod, slightly crushed (optional)

- Melt butter over medium heat in a 3- or 4-quart heavy saucepan with a tight-fitting lid. Add the dry rice and the shredded coconut and stir to coat. Add coconut milk, water, and salt to the saucepan. Bring the pot to a boil over medium-high heat, then immediately turn the heat to low and simmer the rice, covered, for approximately 40 minutes or more, until the coconut milk and water have been fully absorbed.
- Remove from the heat, and set aside, covered, until meal time. Fluff with a fork and remove cardamom pod before serving.

Servings: 6

Nutrition Facts

Nutrition (per serving): 332 calories, 18.8g total fat, 209mg sodium, 42.8g carbohydrates, 3.2g fiber, 4.5g protein.

Recipe Tips

Basmati rice turns out especially well if the rice is soaked for 30 minutes, then drained and rinsed, before proceeding with the recipe.

Asian Cucumber Salad

An Asian twist on marinated cucumbers.

1 large cucumber, peeled and cut into match sticks
2 tablespoons rice wine vinegar
1 teaspoon granulated sugar, or more to taste
1 tablespoon reduced-sodium soy sauce
1 teaspoon sesame oil
½ cup grape tomatoes, halved

- Combine all ingredients in a ceramic dish and chill for 2 hours. Stir occasionally to distribute marinade evenly.
- Serve cold.

Servings: 5

Nutrition Facts

Nutrition (per serving): 24 calories, 1g total fat, 122mg sodium, 5.6g carbohydrates, <1g fiber, <1g protein.

Classic Potato Salad

Serve this dish so freshly prepared that it is still slightly warm—it practically melts in your mouth.

2 pounds potatoes
2 hard boiled eggs, diced
1 cup cucumber, peeled and diced
¼ cup chives, snipped
½ cup radishes, sliced
2 tablespoons filtered cider vinegar
⅔ cup real mayonnaise
½ teaspoon salt
½ teaspoon black pepper, freshly ground

- Scrub and cube the potatoes into bite-sized pieces, leaving the skins on. Cover with water in a medium saucepan and bring to a boil. Turn down heat and simmer until tender, approximately 20 minutes. Drain, sprinkle with cider vinegar, and set aside to cool.
- Combine mayonnaise, salt, and pepper in a large bowl and stir until smooth. Add the cooled or still slightly warm potatoes, diced eggs, cucumbers, chives, and radishes, and toss to coat.
- Serve immediately while slightly warm, or store in refrigerator until serving.

Servings: 6

Nutrition Facts

Nutrition (per serving): 370 calories, 21.6g total fat, 374mg sodium, 39g carbohydrates, 3.9g fiber, 6.6g protein.

Recipe Tips

If substituting potatoes with heavy skins, peel them before cubing.

Company Mashed Potatoes

As the title indicates, these are not your everyday mashed potatoes. These are extra special, and the recipe serves a crowd.

4 cups cooked and mashed potatoes (6-8 potatoes)
2 cups lactose-free cottage cheese
1 cup sour cream
2 tablespoons garlic-infused extra virgin olive oil
2 tablespoons chives, snipped
2 teaspoons salt
⅛ teaspoon white pepper
½ cup Cheddar cheese, grated
¼ cup butter, melted

- Preheat oven to 350° F. Grease a 9" by 13" baking dish with butter and set aside.
- Combine the first 8 ingredients in a large pot or bowl. Transfer potato mixture to the baking dish and spread out with the back of a spoon. Drizzle the potatoes with melted butter.
- Bake for 45 minutes or until heated through and golden brown on the edges. Serve hot.

Servings: 10

Nutrition Facts

Nutrition (per serving): 343 calories, 17.3g total fat, 624mg sodium, 36.8g carbohydrates, 3.5g fiber, 11.3g protein.

Potato Latkes

Latkes, or potato pancakes, are a traditional Hanukkah food, delicious served with a dab of sour cream.

3 medium russet potatoes, peeled and grated on large holes of a box grater
2 tablespoons chives, snipped
½ teaspoon salt
¼ teaspoon black pepper, freshly ground
1 large egg
2 tablespoons olive oil

- Preheat oven to 200° F.
- Squeeze excess water out of the grated potatoes by pressing them in a colander, potato ricer, or tortilla press.
- Stir together potatoes, chives, salt, pepper, and egg whites.
- Heat 1 tablespoon of hot oil over medium heat in a non-stick skillet until oil is shimmering and fragrant. Drop half the potato mixture by spoonfuls into 6 pancakes. Flatten into disks. Cook on each side for approximately 5-7 minutes until golden brown. Remove the latkes to an oven-proof dish and hold, uncovered, in the warm oven while cooking the second batch.
- Serve warm.

Servings: 6

Nutrition Facts

Nutrition (per serving): 114 calories, 5.3g total fat, 209mg sodium, 14.7g carbohydrates, 1.1g fiber, 2.6g protein.

Recipe Tips

The trick to perfect latkes is getting the grated potatoes as dry as possible before combining with the other ingredients. A potato ricer, which is usually used to process cooked potatoes, does a terrific job putting the squeeze on the raw grated potatoes. If no pressing tools are available, wring the grated potatoes in a clean dish towel.

Maple Butternut Squash Casserole

Is this a side dish or a dessert? You decide.

> ¼ **cup stone-ground cornmeal**
> 1 ½ **cup lactose-free milk**
> 2 **tablespoons butter**
> ⅓ **cup 100% pure maple syrup**
> 2 **cups butternut squash, cooked and mashed**
> ½ **teaspoon salt**
> ½ **teaspoon cinnamon**
> ¼ **teaspoon nutmeg**
> ½ **teaspoon ground black pepper**
> 2 **large eggs**

- Preheat oven to 350° F and grease a 2-quart casserole dish with butter or cooking spray.
- Place cornmeal in 2-quart saucepan, add milk, and bring to a boil, stirring constantly. Cool the milk mixture before proceeding. Add the remaining ingredients and stir to mix thoroughly. Spoon into the greased casserole dish.
- Bake for 45 minutes. Remove the casserole from the oven and serve immediately.

Servings: 8

Nutrition Facts

Nutrition (per serving): 129 calories, 4.4g total fat, 187mg sodium, 19.9g carbohydrates, <1g fiber, 4g protein.

Seven Layer Salad

Prepare and serve Seven Layer Salad in a glass salad bowl or trifle dish so each layer can be seen and appreciated. This recipe was so good for last summer's entertaining that I had to "test" it several times.

> 1 ½ **cup mayonnaise**
> 2 **tablespoons granulated sugar**
> 1 **tablespoon white vinegar**
> 1 **large head red leaf lettuce, torn in pieces**
> 4 **hard boiled eggs, sliced**
> 1 **cup carrots, shredded**
> 1 **large green bell pepper, diced**
> ½ **pounds reduced sodium bacon, cooked, drained, and crumbled**
> 2 **cups Cheddar cheese, shredded**

- Combine mayonnaise, vinegar, and sugar in a small bowl and set aside.
- Place each of the remaining ingredients in successive layers in an extra large glass serving bowl. Drizzle the mayonnaise dressing over the salad and refrigerate until chilled or up to 24 hours.
- Toss the salad immediately before serving.

Servings: 12

Nutrition Facts

Nutrition (per serving): 181 calories, 12g total fat, 346mg sodium, 10.4g carbohydrates, 2.1g fiber, 8.6g protein.

Recipe Tips

This recipe was tested with Hellman's mayonnaise. You can substitute ½ cup of lactose-free yogurt for an equal amount of mayonnaise if you prefer.

Oven-Baked French Fries

This easy treatment works just as well with sweet potatoes.

3 medium potatoes
1 tablespoon olive oil
¼ teaspoon paprika
¼ teaspoon salt
Black pepper, freshly ground (optional)

- Preheat oven to 450° F.
- Scrub or peel potatoes. Halve potatoes lengthwise and slice into ½-inch thick strips. Arrange potato strips in a single layer on an uninsulated baking sheet. Drizzle them with oil and stir to coat. Sprinkle with paprika, salt, and pepper, if desired.
- Bake for 30-40 minutes, until potatoes are tender and golden brown.

Servings: 6

Nutrition Facts

Nutrition (per serving): 102 calories, 2.4g total fat, 103mg sodium, 18.7g carbohydrates, 2.4g fiber, 2.2g protein.

Polenta

Polenta doesn't have to come from a tube at the grocery store. This version of polenta cooks up quickly compared to more traditional recipes, which call for more water and far more stirring. This inexpensive and delicious side dish is ready in 15 minutes or less.

3 cups water
½ teaspoon salt
1 cup coarsely ground cornmeal
1 tablespoon butter
⅛ teaspoon red pepper flakes (optional)
½ cup Parmesan cheese, grated

- Bring the water and salt to a boil in a medium saucepan. Add the cornmeal in a thin, steady stream while whisking briskly. Stir in the butter and optional crushed red pepper. Turn the heat down to low and simmer for 5-10 minutes or until thickened. Polenta sputters as it cooks, so cover the pan when you are not stirring it. Remove from the heat, stir in the cheese, and serve.

Servings: 4

Nutrition Facts

Nutrition (per serving): 190 calories, 7.6g total fat, 498mg sodium, 24g carbohydrates, 2.2g fiber, 7.3g protein.

Recipe Tips

Polenta sets up as it cools. For a change of pace, spread hot polenta in a buttered pie plate, top with some FODMAP-friendly vegetables and cheese, and bake your polenta "pizza" until it's heated through.

Warm Potato and Green Bean Salad

Easy and full of flavor. I can't wait to serve this again.

> **3 pounds thin-skinned potatoes, scrubbed and cut into uniform pieces**
> **10-ounces package frozen green beans**
> **3 tablespoons balsamic vinegar**
> **1 tablespoon country style Dijon mustard**
> **⅓ cup extra virgin olive oil**
> **½ teaspoon sea salt**
> **¼ cup fresh parsley, chopped**

- Place potatoes in a large pot of water, cover, and bring to a boil over high heat. Reduce heat to low. Simmer for 10-15 minutes until tender. For the last 2-4 minutes of cooking (depending on the size of your green beans) add the frozen green beans. Remove from heat, drain immediately, and transfer to a serving bowl.
- In a small bowl, combine vinegar, Dijon mustard, olive oil, salt, and fresh parsley. Drizzle the dressing over the potatoes and serve immediately.

> Servings: 6

Nutrition Facts

Nutrition (per serving): 305 calories, 12.5g total fat, 245mg sodium, 47.9g carbohydrates, 5.1g fiber, 5.8g protein.

Recipe Tips

10 ounces of fresh green beans, cooked, can be substituted for frozen beans.
This recipe was tested with Grey Poupon Country Style Dijon mustard.

Roasted Carrots

Roasted vegetables are usually served as a side dish at dinner, but why not make extra to enjoy with tomorrow's eggs or green salad?

> **1 pound carrots, peeled and cut into sticks of uniform size**
> **1 tablespoon olive oil or garlic-infused oil**
> **1 teaspoon whole-grain mustard**
> **¼ teaspoon salt**
> **1 teaspoon 100% pure maple syrup**
> **¼ teaspoon black pepper, freshly ground**

- Preheat oven to 475° F.
- Distribute the prepared carrots on a large baking tray. Combine oil, mustard, salt, and maple syrup in a small bowl and drizzle over the carrots. Roast the carrots until tender, approximately 20 minutes, stirring once or twice. Small pieces that seem in danger of burning can be removed to a serving dish as needed.

> Servings: 4

Nutrition Facts

Nutrition (per serving): 82 calories, 3.8g total fat, 240mg sodium, 12.2g carbohydrates, 3.2g fiber, 1.2g protein.

Recipe Tips

Many other vegetables can be roasted in a similar fashion. Try roasted zucchini, sweet potatoes, white potatoes, parsnips, fennel bulb, or butternut squash.

Soups and Stews

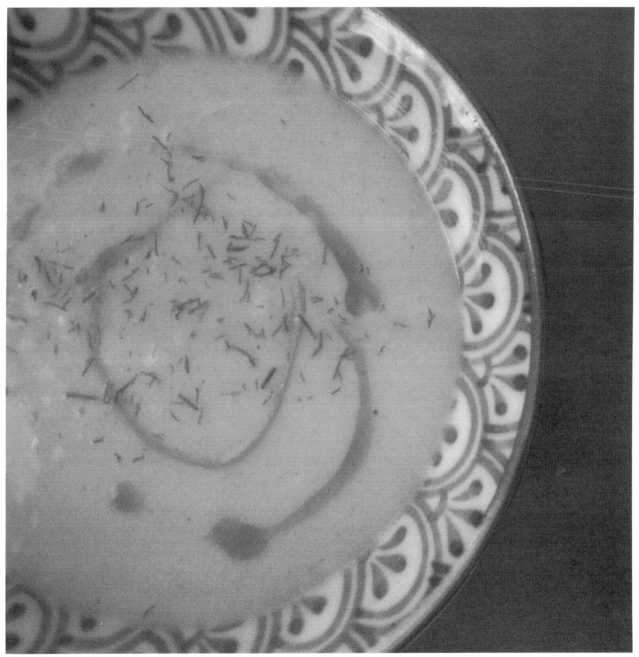

Avgolemono Soup

Avgolemono Soup

The Greek community in our city holds a fabulous Greek Festival each June. We make a point of going to celebrate my husband's Greek heritage. I adapted this recipe from one I found in the community cookbook sold at the festival. The egg turns the broth a creamy yellow color.

> **6 medium boneless chicken thighs**
> **8 cups water**
> **1 Bouquet Garni (recipe)**
> **½ cup short or medium grain rice, white or brown**
> **3 large eggs, lightly beaten**
> **1 teaspoon salt**
> **½ teaspoon black pepper, freshly ground**
> **juice of two small lemons**
> **½ cup parsley, chopped**

- Bring chicken, water, and Bouquet Garni to a boil in an 8-quart soup kettle. Reduce heat and simmer until chicken is fully cooked, approximately 20 minutes, then remove from heat.
- When chicken is cool enough to handle, remove pieces from the chicken broth. Pull meat off the bone and shred into bite-sized pieces. Set aside. Discard the Bouquet Garni but reserve the chicken broth.
- Add the rice to the chicken broth in the saucepan, bring to a boil over high heat, then reduce heat to low and simmer for 30 minutes or until rice is tender.
- Meanwhile, beat the eggs until fluffy in a large bowl using an electric mixer or hand whisk. Add lemon juice to the eggs slowly while mixing. Add the hot broth to this mixture a little bit at a time, beating constantly, until you have used up about half the broth. Return the egg mixture to the remaining broth in the soup pot, stirring constantly. Add the chicken meat, salt and pepper to the soup and heat it to at least 180° F, but do not boil.
- Adjust seasonings and garnish with fresh parsley or curls of lemon rind, if desired. Serve immediately.

> Servings: 6

Nutrition Facts

Nutrition (per serving): 208 calories, 8.0g total fat, 475mg sodium, 15.2g carbohydrates, <1g fiber, 18.2g protein.

Recipe Tips

Warming up the eggs with broth before adding them to the soup pot prevents them from curdling.
If you have some frozen Chicken Stock on hand to use in place of water, the meat from a grocery store rotisserie chicken can be used for this recipe.

Basic Chicken Stock

Commercial stocks or broth almost always contain onions, garlic, or other objectionable ingredients. Yours will have these flavors, too, but by removing the flesh of the onions and garlic before adding water, you will be subtracting the FODMAPs.

> **1 small onion, peeled and quartered**
> **1 clove garlic, slightly crushed but still intact**
> **2 tablespoons garlic-infused olive oil**
> **8 cups boiling water**
> **1 pound chicken skin-on or skinless drumsticks**
> **1 fresh tomato, diced**
> **2 carrots, scrubbed and coarsely chopped**
> **Bouquet Garni (recipe)**
> **10 peppercorns**
> **1 teaspoon salt (optional)**

- Heat olive oil, garlic, and onion together in a large stock pot over medium heat. When onions are translucent, remove the onion and garlic from the pot and discard, leaving the flavored oil in the pot. Add the remaining ingredients. Reduce heat, and allow to simmer, covered, for 1 hour.
- Cool briefly, then strain the stock through a sieve into a clean container.
- If desired, remove the meat from the chicken bones and return to the broth or reserve for another use, discarding the bones, skin, and vegetables.
- Use immediately or refrigerate for up to 3 days.

    Servings: 7, 1 cup each
    Yield: 7 cups

Nutrition Facts

Nutrition (per serving): 157 calories, 9.6g total fat, 411mg sodium, 4.2g carbohydrates, 1.1g fiber, 13g protein.

Recipe Tips

If desired, hardened fat may be easily removed from the top of the refrigerated broth.
Stock freezes well. Pour into freezer safe containers, allowing some headroom for expansion, and freeze.
Nutrition information for this recipe includes the chicken meat and the optional salt.

East Indies Green Soup

This fragrant and colorful soup pairs well with thick slices of warm Basic Yeast Bread (recipe). With its bright greens and reds, it will look wonderful on a holiday table or buffet. Or make it on a chilly Sunday evening and bring the leftovers for lunch during the week.

2 tablespoons garlic-infused extra virgin olive oil
2 tablespoons ginger root, peeled and minced
1 teaspoon sugar
1 teaspoon sea salt, or more to taste
¼ teaspoon ground turmeric
¼ teaspoon ground allspice
¼ teaspoon ground nutmeg
1 pinch cayenne pepper (optional)
2 medium potatoes, peeled, cubed
4 cups zucchini, diced
4 cups Chicken Stock or water
1 cup chicken pieces
1 cup fresh spinach, chopped
½ red bell pepper, seeded and diced

- Heat the garlic-infused oil in an 8-quart stock pot until fragrant. Stir in the ginger and spices and cook for 5 minutes. Add potatoes, zucchini, and chicken stock. Bring to a boil, reduce heat to low, and simmer for 20 minutes or until potatoes are tender.
- Remove soup from heat, adjust seasonings, and stir in the spinach. Using a stick blender, blend soup until smooth.
- Stir in chicken pieces and transfer soup to bowls. Serve garnished with red bell pepper.

    Servings: 6

Nutrition Facts

Nutrition (per serving): 143 calories, 6.3g total fat, 351mg sodium, 14.6g carbohydrates, 2g fiber, 8.2g protein.

Recipe Tips

Nutrients were calculated using water for liquid, but the flavor is extra special if you use homemade Chicken Stock.

Italian Wedding Soup

Meatball soup with greens. Nothing fancy, but easy and filling, this is one of those recipes you can make on Sunday evening and enjoy for lunch over the next couple of days.

12 ounces ground turkey or beef
1 large egg
2 tablespoons quick cooking oats
1 teaspoon Parmesan cheese, grated
½ teaspoon dried basil
2 teaspoons garlic-infused oil
3 ½ cups Chicken Stock (recipe) or water
2 medium carrots, peeled and diced
½ cup brown rice, uncooked
4 cups Swiss chard, chopped

- Combine ground turkey, egg, oats, Parmesan cheese, and basil in a mixing bowl. Form into 1" balls, using your hands or a small scoop.
- Heat the olive oil in a non-stick skillet over medium heat until fragrant. Brown the meatballs and drain excess fat.
- In a large saucepan, bring chicken broth to a boil. Stir in carrots, meatballs, and rice. Cover the pot and simmer until both carrots and rice are tender. Add the Swiss chard and cook briefly until leaves are wilted. Add salt and pepper, if desired.
- Garnish with Parmesan cheese.

Servings: 4

Nutrition Facts

Nutrition (per serving): 347 calories, 13.9g total fat, 465mg sodium, 32.7g carbohydrates, 3.3g fiber, 24g protein.

Gazpacho

I learned to make gazpacho as a child, using fresh tomatoes from my mother's garden. It's been one of my favorites ever since.

1 cup water
4 large fresh tomatoes, cut into wedges, or a 28-ounce can of diced tomatoes
¼ cup red wine vinegar
2 tablespoons garlic-infused extra virgin olive oil
1 medium cucumber, peeled and cut into 1-inch slices
1 medium green bell pepper, seeded and diced
¾ teaspoon salt
¼ teaspoon pepper
¼ cup chives, snipped
½ teaspoon dried oregano
½ teaspoon red pepper flakes (optional)
2 tablespoons sour cream

- Place all ingredients (except sour cream) in the bowl of a blender or food processor in the order listed. Chop to the desired consistency. Stir in chives.
- Chill until serving. Divide into serving bowls and garnish with a dab of sour cream.

Servings: 5

Nutrition Facts

Nutrition (per serving): 98 calories, 6.8g total fat, 363mg sodium, 8.5g carbohydrates, 2.7g fiber, 2g protein.

Mom's Fish Chowder

This chowder always hits the spot and takes less than an hour to make.

3 tablespoons butter
½ cup carrots, peeled and diced
1 small onion, peeled and quartered
4 large potatoes (about 2 pounds), peeled and cubed
1 bay leaf
1 ½ pounds cod or haddock
1 quart lactose-free whole milk
½ teaspoon salt
¼ teaspoon black pepper, freshly ground

- Melt butter in a large soup kettle over medium heat. Add carrots and onions and sauté until tender, approximately 5-10 minutes. Remove the onions.
- Add potatoes, bay leaf, and just enough water to barely cover the potatoes. Cover the pot and bring to a boil over medium-high heat. Turn down heat and simmer until potatoes are tender, about 15 minutes. Remove the bay leaf. Lay the raw fish filet across the top of the potatoes. Cover pot and continue to simmer until the fish is opaque and flakes apart easily. Use a fork to break up the fish into bite-sized pieces.
- Add the milk, salt, and pepper, then warm the chowder gently until the milk is heated through; do not boil. Adjust seasonings and serve immediately, or refrigerate to be warmed gently the next day.

Servings: 6

Nutrition Facts

Nutrition (per serving): 404 calories, 11.9g total fat, 385mg sodium, 45.6g carbohydrates, 3.1g fiber, 29.5g protein.

Slow Cooker Beef Stew

For consistently tender stew, purchase a chuck roast and cut it up at home instead of buying prepared an unknown cut labeled "stew meat." Your stew will be ready to serve when you get home from work.

1 tablespoon olive oil or garlic-infused oil
2 pounds chuck roast, cut into large bite-sized pieces
¼ cup brown rice flour
1 teaspoon salt
½ teaspoon ground black pepper
Bouquet Garni (recipe)
3 large carrots, peeled and quartered
2 large potatoes, peeled and cut into 1-inch cubes
1 cup water

- Measure the oil into a 2- or 3-quart slow cooker.
- Add the cubed stew meat and stir to coat. Sprinkle the rice flour, salt, and pepper over the meat, and again stir to coat. Add the Bouquet Garni, vegetables, and water into the slow cooker. Cover and cook undisturbed on low for 8 hours.
- Stir and remove Bouquet Garni before serving.

Servings: 5

Nutrition Facts

Nutrition (per serving): 510 calories, 14.5g total fat, 584mg sodium, 25.8g carbohydrates, 2.7g fiber, 66g protein.

Recipe Tips

If using a larger slow cooker, you may have to adjust the amount of liquid and the cooking time accordingly.

No-Bean Chili Soup

Garnish mugs of this chili with sour cream, shredded Cheddar, and sliced scallion greens or chives. It makes a large batch, suitable for a Super Bowl party or potluck dinner.

> **2 pounds lean ground beef**
> **1 medium green bell pepper, diced**
> **1 medium red bell pepper, diced**
> **1 small fennel bulb, diced**
> **1 small Serrano or jalapeno pepper, chopped (optional)**
> **2 tablespoons ground chili powder**
> **2 tablespoons ground cumin**
> **2 teaspoons dried oregano**
> **1 teaspoon salt**
> **1 tablespoon granulated sugar**
> **1 (28-ounce) can diced tomatoes with liquid**
> **1 cup water**

- Sauté the ground beef in a large skillet over medium heat. Crumble the meat into bite-sized pieces as it cooks. When the meat is no longer pink, remove from heat and drain the fat off. Return the skillet to the heat and add the diced vegetables and optional Serrano or jalapeno pepper. Turn the heat down to low and cook, stirring occasionally, until vegetables are tender. Add the spices, canned tomatoes, and water to the pot and stir.

- Simmer over low heat for 1 ½ hours; serve hot.

> Servings: 8

Nutrition Facts

Nutrition (per serving): 274 calories, 17.6g total fat, 512mg sodium, 9.7g carbohydrates, 2.8g fiber, 19.8g protein.

Desserts

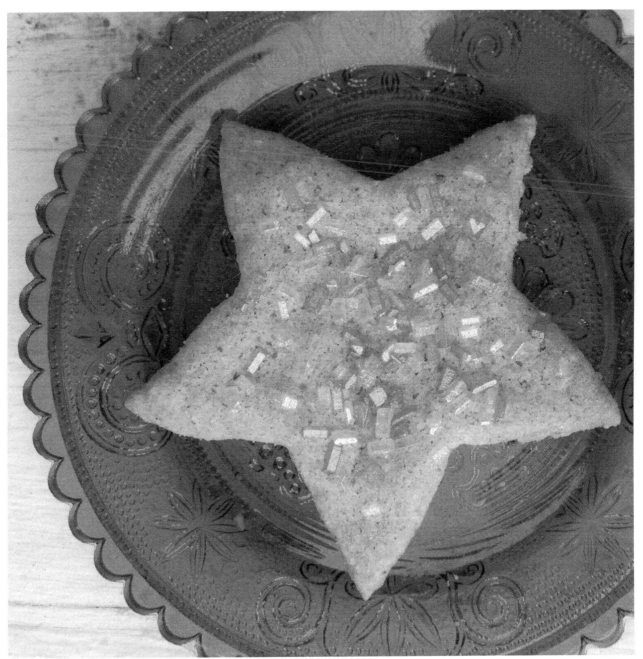

Best Ever Roll-Out Sugar Cookies

Best Roll-Out Sugar Cookies

These sugar cookies are sweet and crispy. The dough handles beautifully and the cookies hold their shape during baking. They stay fresh for days, so you can make them ahead for special holiday occasions.

½ cup butter (no substitutes)
1 cup granulated sugar
2 large egg yolks
1 teaspoon vanilla
1 tablespoon milk
½ teaspoon baking soda
1 cup sweet white sorghum flour
¼ cup brown rice flour
¼ cup tapioca flour
¼ cup almond meal
1 tablespoon ground chia seeds
colored sugar for decorating

- Combine softened butter, sugar, egg yolks, vanilla, and milk in a large mixing bowl, using a wooden spoon. Add the dry ingredients and stir until a stiff uniform dough is formed. If dough is too sticky, add sorghum flour one tablespoon at a time and stir to combine.
- Use clean hands to form two flattened balls of dough. Wrap tightly with plastic wrap and chill dough for at least one hour.
- Preheat over to 350° F.
- Dust a clean counter top and a wooden rolling pin liberally with sorghum flour. Remove one dough ball at a time from the refrigerator, unwrap it, and roll it out to ⅛" thick on the counter top. Use more sorghum flour on top of the dough if it sticks to the rolling pin. Cut out shapes with cookie cutters, sprinkle with colored sugar and transfer to an ungreased cookie sheet using a thin metal spatula. Leave at least ½ inch between cookie shapes.
- Bake for 8 minutes or until edges are beginning to turn golden brown. Remove the cookie sheet from the oven and allow the cookies to cool for 2-3 minutes before using a metal spatula to transfer them to a wire cooling rack. Enjoy immediately or store cooled cookies in an airtight container until serving.

Servings: 36

Nutrition Facts

Nutrition (per serving): 80 calories, 3.6g total fat, 19mg sodium, 11.6g carbohydrates, .6g fiber, 1.1g protein

Tips

The number of servings for this recipe varies depending on the size of the cookie cutters used.
You can substitute 1 ½ cups of King Arthur gluten-free multipurpose flour for the sorghum, brown rice flour, tapioca flour, almond meal, and chia seeds.
Have a little extra on hand for dusting the counter top and rolling pin.

Mini Melon Cups

The trick to keeping fruit IBS-friendly is limiting portion sizes to ½ cup per meal or snack. These fruit cups are just adorable when made with an extra small (½ -inch diameter) melon baller.

2 naval oranges
¼ cantaloupe
¼ honeydew melon
1 bunch fresh mint leaves

- Cut a thin slice off each end of the navel orange to help them stand up securely on a plate without tipping over. Cut the oranges in half and run a serrated knife around the rim of each half, as if you were cutting a grapefruit. Use a melon baller to hollow out the inside of the oranges, reserve the pulp and juice in a glass measuring cup.
- Prepare a total of two cups of miniature cantaloupe and honeydew melon balls. Pour the reserved orange juice over the melon balls, using a fork to hold back the orange pulp. Place the 4 orange halves on a serving plate. Fill each with miniature melon balls and garnish with mint slices.
- Serve chilled.

Servings: 4

Nutrition Facts

Nutrition (per serving): 67 calories, .3g total fat, 18mg sodium, 17.3g carbohydrates, 1.3g fiber, 1.3g protein

Baked Custard

Baked custard is one of life's simple pleasures, and an enjoyable way to increase your protein intake.

3 large eggs
⅓ cup 100% pure maple syrup
1 teaspoon vanilla extract
2 ½ cups lactose-free milk

- Preheat oven to 350° F and put a kettle of water on to boil. Lightly grease 6 glass custard cups with butter or oil and set aside.
- Scald milk in microwave or on stovetop. (Heat until small bubbles form around edges and milk is steaming. Do not boil.) Set aside to cool for about 10 minutes.
- In a separate bowl, whip together eggs, sugar, and vanilla. Very slowly pour warm milk into egg mixture, stirring briskly. Pour the custard mixture into the prepared custard cups and place them in a 2"-deep roasting or baking pan. Pour boiling water into the pan, surrounding the custard cups with at least an inch of water.
- Carefully place the roasting pan in the oven and bake for approximately 45 minutes or until a knife inserted in the center comes out clean. Turn oven off, open oven door slightly, and allow to cool until custard cups can safely be removed from the hot water bath.
- Cover and chill in refrigerator until ready to serve.

Servings: 6

Nutrition Facts

Nutrition (per serving): 132 calories, 5g total fat, 77mg sodium, 16g carbohydrates, 0g fiber, 6g protein.

Peppermint Patty Shake

Peppermint oil is effective at calming the IBS gut, so why not try peppermint in its original form? Fresh peppermint is available year-round at well-stocked conventional or Asian grocery stores or seasonally at your local farmer's market. It has purple, square-shaped stems, and pointier, slightly shinier leaves than its cousin, spearmint. If you have gastroesophageal reflux disease (GERD), consume peppermint with caution.

>   **¾ cup lactose-free milk**
>   **1 cup lactose-free ice cream**
>   **½ cup loosely packed peppermint leaves**
>   **¼ cup Chocolate Syrup (recipe)**
>   **1 serving whey protein powder**

- Place all ingredients in the the bowl of a blender in the order listed. Blend on high until a uniform consistency is reached.
- Serve immediately, garnished with a sprig of mint.

>   Servings: 2

Nutrition Facts

Nutrition (per serving): 288 calories, 8.1g total fat, 128mg sodium, 44.8g carbohydrates, 2.4g fiber, 9.8g protein.

Recipe Tips

This recipe was tested with Breyer's lactose-free vanilla ice cream.

Chocolate Macaroons

Reminiscent of a Mounds Bar, these travel and freeze well, but be sure to try one while they are still warm for melt-in-your-mouth chocolatey goodness.

>   **1 cup egg whites**
>   **⅔ cup sugar**
>   **3 cups unsweetened coconut flakes**
>   **½ teaspoon vanilla**
>   **½ cup miniature semisweet chocolate chips**

- Preheat oven to 300° F. Cover 2 baking trays with parchment paper and set aside.
- Combine egg whites, sugar, and coconut flakes in a 4-quart saucepan. Stir over medium-low heat for 8-12 minutes until the sticky, moist dough suddenly becomes drier. Remove from the heat, stir in vanilla and chocolate chips, cover, and chill in the refrigerator for 30 minutes.
- Use a small scoop to transfer 1-inch balls of dough to the prepared baking trays.
- Bake for 30 minutes. Cookies will be firm to the touch.
- Cool completely on the cookie tray before removing and storing in an airtight container.

>   Servings: 36

Nutrition Facts

Nutrition (per serving): 153 calories, 13g total fat, 20mg sodium, 9g carbohydrates, 3g fiber, 2g protein.

Recipe Tips

It isn't difficult to separate egg whites from the yolks once you've seen how it's done; ask a friend to demonstrate or look for a video on YouTube.

Crustless Kabocha Pie

This one's a keeper!

2 cups kabocha squash, cooked and puréed
2 large eggs
⅓ cup brown sugar, firmly packed
⅓ cup granulated sugar
1 tablespoon cornstarch
½ teaspoon cinnamon
½ teaspoon ginger
½ teaspoon nutmeg
¼ teaspoon salt
1 ½ cups lactose-free milk

- Preheat oven to 350° F and put a kettle of water on to boil. Lightly grease 6 glass custard cups with butter or oil and set aside.
- Combine the squash, eggs, and sugars in a large bowl. Stir in the dry ingredients. Add milk and stir until a smooth and uniform consistency is reached. Pour the kabocha mixture into the prepared custard cups and place them in a 2" deep roasting or baking pan. Pour boiling water in the pan to a depth of at least an inch.
- Carefully place the roasting pan in the oven and bake for approximately 50 minutes. Start checking at 40 minutes. The custard is done when a knife inserted in the center comes out clean. Turn oven off, open oven door slightly, and allow to cool until custard cups can safely be removed from the hot water bath.
- Serve warm, or cover and chill until serving.

Servings: 8

Nutrition Facts

Nutrition (per serving): 174 calories, 2.6g fat, 106mg sodium, 34.4g carbohydrate, 2.5g fiber, 5.1g protein

Recipe Tips

Prepare your kabocha squash for this recipe by cutting it in half and oven-roasting it until tender. When it is cool enough to handle, remove the flesh and purée it in a blender of food processor, adding water as necessary to get a texture similar to canned pumpkin.

Banana "Ice Cream"

It's hard to believe this creamy dessert is almost nothing but fruit.

3 tablespoons water
2 ripe bananas, peeled
½ teaspoon vanilla extract
¼ teaspoon cinnamon
1 ice cube

- Slice banana into ½-inch coins and spread out on a plate. Freeze for 2 hours.
- Place ingredients in the bowl of a blender or food processor and process until creamy.
- Serve immediately or freeze to serve later in the day.

Servings: 4

Nutrition Facts

Nutrition (per serving): 54 calories, <1g total fat, 1mg sodium, 13.7g carbohydrates, 1.6g fiber, <1g protein.

Recipe Tips

For extra calories and richer flavor, use a cube of frozen coconut milk or cream instead of a regular ice cube.

Berry-Ricotta Tart

This delightful tart belongs on the menu whenever fresh berries are available. It's very attractive and adds color to any buffet table.

1 recipe Pecan Shortbread Sand Dollars, uncooked (recipe)
1 ¼ cup ricotta cheese
¼ teaspoon salt
¼ teaspoon cinnamon
3 tablespoons 100% pure maple syrup
2 cups fresh blueberries or raspberries

- Preheat oven to 375° F.
- Press the shortbread dough into the bottom of an unbuttered 9.5" tart pan or springform pan.
- Bake for 25 minutes or until golden brown.
- Remove from oven and cool to room temperature.
- Mix together ricotta cheese, salt, cinnamon, and maple syrup. Spread over the cooled cookie crust. Arrange berries on top. Sprinkle with lemon zest.
- Chill for 2 hours.
- Just before serving, drizzle with a little additional maple syrup.

Servings: 8

Nutrition Facts

Nutrition (per serving): 375 calories, 21.9g total fat, 126mg sodium, 37.3g carbohydrates, 3.3g fiber, 9.5g protein.

Chocolate Pudding

Pudding is delicious, comforting, and easily made FODMAP-friendly with the use of lactose-free milk.

½ cup granulated sugar
5 tablespoons cornstarch
¼ cup cocoa powder
3 cups lactose-free milk
2 teaspoons vanilla extract
⅛ teaspoon salt

- Stir sugar, cornstarch, and cocoa powder together in a medium saucepan until thoroughly combined. Gradually whisk in the milk and vanilla. If necessary, work out any lumps of cornstarch with the back of a spoon.
- Cook over medium-low heat, stirring constantly until the pudding thickens. Remove from heat just before the pudding begins to boil.
- Cover and chill. Serve cold.

Servings: 6

Nutrition Facts

Nutrition (per serving): 163 calories, 2.9g total fat, 100mg sodium, 31g carbohydrates, 1.g fiber, 4.8g protein.

Recipe Tips

This recipe was tested with Ghirardelli cocoa powder.

Crispy Rice Treats

This sweet and crunchy classic will be enjoyed by young and old at your next party.

3 tablespoons butter
1 package (10 ounces) marshmallows
6 cups crispy rice cereal

- Butter a 9" by 13" baking dish and set aside.
- Melt the butter over low heat in an 8-quart saucepan. Add marshmallows and stir until completely melted. Remove from heat and stir in crispy rice cereal. Using a buttered spatula or buttered fingertips, press the mixture evenly into the baking pan.
- Cool and cut into squares. Store in an air-tight container.

Servings: 12

Nutrition Facts

Nutrition (per serving): 151 calories, 3.1g total fat, 145mg sodium, 31g carbohydrates, <1g fiber, 1.4g protein.

Recipe Tips

For special occasions, pack the crispy rice mixture into buttered cookie cutters to form hearts or other shapes.

Lemon Squares

Oh my, these are good. The Pecan Shortbread crust paired with the sweet-tart lemon custard is a match made in heaven.

1 recipe Pecan Shortbread Sand Dollars, uncooked
2 tablespoons lemon juice concentrate
3 large eggs
1 ½ cups sugar
1 tablespoon cornstarch
1 ½ teaspoons baking powder
1 pinch salt

- Preheat the oven to 350° F.
- Press the Pecan Shortbread dough across the bottom of an ungreased 9" by 9" baking dish and bake for 35 minutes.
- Meanwhile, place the remaining ingredients in a medium-sized mixing bowl and beat for 3 minutes with an electric mixer on medium-high. Pour over the hot crust and return the baking dish to the oven.
- Bake for 20 minutes, then reduce heat to 300° F for another 10 minutes. Lemon custard will still be soft when done, but should not appear to be runny when the baking dish is tilted. It will have a golden brown crust, somewhat browner on the edges.

Servings: 12

Nutrition Facts

Nutrition (per serving): 306 calories, 13.7g total fat, 105mg sodium, 42.7g carbohydrates, 1.6g fiber, 4.8g protein.

Recipe Tips

The recipe was tested with ReaLemon 100% lemon juice from concentrate. Juice made *from* lemon juice concentrated is fine, even though fruit juice concentrates used as sweeteners in some processed foods are not recommended.

Magic Coconut Pie

This is an example of a recipe that is easily adapted to wheat-free baking because the original recipe called for very little flour in the first place. This attractive pie will be welcome on any buffet table. It magically forms a crust on the bottom as it bakes.

    3 large eggs
    1 ¼ cups lactose-free milk
    1 ¼ cups sugar
    2 tablespoons brown rice flour
    2 tablespoons cornstarch
    2 tablespoons tapioca flour
    1 teaspoon vinegar
    6 tablespoons melted butter
    1 teaspoon vanilla extract
    1 ½ cups coconut flakes, unsweetened

- Preheat the oven to 325° F. Lightly grease a 9″ pie plate with butter or oil and set aside.
- Beat eggs, milk, and sugar together in a medium-sized bowl. Add remaining ingredients and mix thoroughly. Transfer the mixture to the prepared pie plate.
- Bake for 35-40 minutes until golden brown and bubbly on the edges.
- Chill for several hours or overnight before serving.

    Servings: 10

Nutrition Facts

Nutrition (per serving): 401 calories, 27.1g total fat, 94mg sodium, 38.1g carbohydrates, 4.7g fiber, 5.1g protein.

Maple-Walnut Brittle

You need a candy thermometer for this one. This recipe is not suitable for making with young children. The candy gets extremely hot and could cause a serious burn.

    2 cups walnut pieces
    ¼ cup 100% pure maple syrup
    1 cup granulated sugar
    1 cup butter
    ¼ cup water

- Stir walnuts in a heavy, ungreased frying pan over medium-high heat with a wooden spoon until fragrant and slightly toasted. Watch closely, as nuts burn easily. Set aside.
- Stir together syrup, sugar, butter, and water in a clean, heavy-bottomed, 4-quart saucepan until melted and creamy. Clip the candy thermometer on the side of the saucepan. Be sure the thermometer is not resting on the bottom of the saucepan. Bring the mixture to a gentle boil over medium heat and *do not stir again* until the candy thermometer reaches 300° F (hard crack stage). This may take 15-20 minutes. Don't rush it by turning up the heat or the candy may scorch. Immediately stir in walnuts.
- Carefully pour the hot mixture onto an ungreased cookie sheet. Use a silicone scraper to empty the bowl and spread the candy out. Cool completely. Break into large pieces and store in an airtight container.

    Servings: 16

Nutrition Facts

Nutrition (per serving): 259 calories, 21.1g total fat, 82mg sodium, 17.9g carbohydrates, <1g fiber, 2.4g protein.

Peanut Brittle

Like the maple-walnut brittle, this is an adults-only project. The sugar syrup gets very hot. Even though it looks delicious, do not lick the spoon.

> **1 cup granulated sugar**
> **½ cup light corn syrup**
> **1 ½ cups oil-roasted, salted peanuts**
> **1 teaspoon butter**
> **1 teaspoon vanilla extract**
> **1 teaspoon baking soda**

- Stir together sugar and corn syrup in a 1-quart microwave safe container. A bowl or extra large measuring cup with a handle would be ideal for safe handling.
- Microwave on high for 4 minutes. Mixture will be extremely hot. Stir in peanuts and microwave on high for 3 minutes more minutes. Add butter and vanilla, blending well. Microwave on high for 1 minute more. Add baking soda and stir until foaminess begins to die down, about 25 strokes.
- Carefully pour the hot mixture onto an ungreased cookie sheet. Use a silicone scraper to empty the bowl and spread the candy out. Cool completely. Break into large pieces and store in an airtight container.

Servings: 12

Nutrition Facts

Nutrition (per serving): 216 calories, 9.8g total fat, 171mg sodium, 30.4g carbohydrates, 1.7g fiber, 5.1g protein.

Recipe Tips

This recipe was tested in a full-sized, 1100-watt microwave oven.

Peanut Butter Fudge

A small piece of this fudge will satisfy your sweet tooth in a most delicious way.

> **1 cup butter**
> **1 pound natural peanut butter**
> **1 teaspoon vanilla**
> **1 pound confectioner's sugar**

- Line an 8" by 8" baking pan with waxed paper.
- Microwave butter and peanut butter together in large microwave-safe mixing bowl until melted. Stir and check every 45 seconds until melted and smooth.
- Add vanilla and confectioner's sugar to peanut butter mixture and stir to combine. Mixture should resemble a thick cookie dough. Add more powdered sugar if necessary to achieve the desired consistency.
- Spoon the fudge into the baking pan and spread out to the edges with a knife or spatula.
- Cover and chill. Cut into 1-inch square pieces and store in an airtight container for up to a week.

Servings: 64

Nutrition Facts

Nutrition (per serving): 94 calories, 6.5g total fat, 53mg sodium, 8.5g carbohydrates, .4g fiber, 1.8g protein.

Recipe Tips

This recipe was tested with Trader Joe's natural, unsalted peanut butter.

Pecan Shortbread Sand Dollars

Not only a great cookie, this recipe makes a wonderful shortbread crust for your favorite bar cookie or fruit tart.

½ cup unsalted butter
1 cup oat flour, loosely packed
1 cup finely ground pecan flour
½ cup granulated sugar
1 egg
1 teaspoon vanilla extract
1 teaspoon pure almond extract

- Preheat oven to 300° F.
- Place butter in a medium-sized, microwave safe mixing bowl; microwave for 15-30 seconds to soften the butter. Add remaining ingredients and stir together with a wooden spoon until a soft dough is formed.
- Drop heaping teaspoons of dough onto ungreased cookie sheets.
- Bake for 20-30 minutes, until golden brown on the edges and firm to the touch.
- Remove from the oven, and use a spatula to transfer the cookies to a paper towel-topped counter. Allow cookies to cool for 30 minutes, then store in an airtight container.

Servings: 12, 2 cookies each; yield 2 dozen

Nutrition Facts

Nutrition (per serving): 193 calories, 12.9g total fat, 9mg sodium, 16.7g carbohydrates, 1.6g fiber, 3.8g protein.

Recipe Tips

Pecan flour can be hard to find. You can grind your own in small batches in your food processor or blender.

Peppermint Meringue Cookies

Light as air, these cookies have a nice retro vibe. Meringue cookies melt in your mouth.

2 large egg whites
¾ cup granulated sugar
⅛ teaspoon cream of tartar
⅛ teaspoon salt
¼ cup crushed Starlight peppermint candies or candy canes

- Beat egg whites with an electric mixer until stiff peaks are formed. Gradually add sugar, cream of tartar, and salt, with mixer running on low speed. Gently stir in crushed candy.
- Drop small spoonfuls on 2 cookie trays lined with parchment paper.
- Bake at 275° F for 25 minutes. Turn off oven. Cool for 2 hours in the oven with the door closed. Store in airtight container.

Servings: 15, 2 cookies each

Nutrition Facts

Nutrition (per serving): 54 calories, 1.3g total fat, 26mg sodium, 10.3g carbohydrates, <1g fiber, <1g protein.

Recipe Tips

Parchment paper is available at your grocery store, shelved with plastic wraps and foils.

Tapioca Pudding

It's a simple, classic treat.

3 cups lactose-free milk
½ cup minute tapioca
½ cup granulated sugar
¼ teaspoon salt
2 large eggs, beaten
1 teaspoon vanilla extract

- Stir together the milk, tapioca, sugar, and salt in a heavy-bottomed saucepan. Bring the mixture to a boil over medium heat, stirring constantly. Pudding has a tendency to scorch, so stirring across the bottom of the pan with a spatula is recommended.

- Remove the mixture from the heat. Add 2 tablespoons of hot milk mixture at a time into the beaten eggs, stirring briskly, in a separate bowl. Continue adding 2 tablespoons of milk at a time until 1 cup of hot milk mixture has been added to eggs. Stir egg mixture back into the tapioca until well mixed.

- Return the mixture to medium-low heat; cook and stir until pudding comes to a gentle simmer and coats the back of a spoon. Stir in vanilla. Garnish with a dash of cinnamon or freshly grated nutmeg if desired. Serve hot or cold.

Servings: 6

Nutrition Facts

Nutrition (per serving): 187 calories, 2.8g total fat, 174mg sodium, 34.2g carbohydrates, <1g fiber, 6.2g protein.

ACKNOWLEDGEMENTS

I began actively working on this cookbook as soon as the first edition of *IBS— Free at Last!* was published in 2009. I've learned it takes a lot of time to develop and test recipes that are worthy of being included in a cookbook, and it is a job that cannot be done alone. For assistance in the kitchen with recipe testing, I'd like to thank my daughter, Laura Catsos, who tested many of these recipes during the winter and spring of 2011. Her assistance was invaluable. Jillian Smith, a dietetics student at the University of New Hampshire, developed and tested several of the recipes in the collection. Most recently, Christine Beecher has assisted me with recipe testing and photography.

Where would a recipe developer be without willing tasters? In that regard my family was always there for me, including Paul, Michael, Christine, and Laura Catsos, and Nicole Proctor-Smith. My extended family cheerfully allowed me to turn every family gathering and vacation over the last few years into a recipe testing occasion. Friends of the family, too numerous to mention, also indulged me as I fed them my creations. Sharon Elizabeth, thanks for reading my manuscript and helping me bring it on home.

I'd like to thank my mother, Suzanne Danehy, for teaching me how to cook. In addition to being an adventurous cook and role model in the kitchen, she served as the cooking teacher for our 4-H club during my preteen years. Later, my work as a short-order cook at the Cascade Diner in Canton, New York, and my four years at Cornell Dining built confidence in the kitchen. I extend my appreciation to those chefs, cooks, and kitchen workers who mentored me. I also benefited from formal instruction in the chemistry of cooking as a nutrition undergraduate at Cornell. My roommates teased me a bit when my final project for one class was baking a series of blueberry pies in pursuit of the flakiest bottom crust. Problem solving in the kitchen has turned out to be a useful professional skill for me after all, so I can claim the last laugh.

I treasure my nutrition colleagues at Nutrition Works, LLC, in Portland, Maine, who continue to inspire me with their dedication to excellent patient care: Susan Quimby, Judy Donnelly, Kim Norbert, and Marissa Stanley. I'd like to thank Susan, in particular, for supporting my work outside the practice, even when it means being away a little more than I would like.

Fellow dietitians Kate Scarlata , Marlisa Brown, and Carol Ireton-Jones: I am proud to have shared the podium or microphone with each of you at workshops and webinars over the past few year. I couldn't be in better company. The "What Every RD Needs to Know About FODMAPs" workshop series has been a blast, and I have enjoyed meeting dietitians all over the country. I appreciate the participation and contributions of each and every attendee and your willingness to share with each other as we build our FODMAP knowledge base and skills together.

As always, I am indebted to my readers, especially those who interact with me on my blog, www.ibsfree.net, on Twitter (CatsosIBSFreeRD), on Pinterest (pcatsos), and on Facebook (IBSFree). Without your encouragement, I would find it far less rewarding to do this work. Some of you have been waiting for this cookbook for rather a long time, and I hope you will not be disappointed. Lauren Pulver, thanks for being a reader extraordinaire and for sharing the stage with me at #140YOU in New York City. Lisa Braithwaite and Erin Cox, you've been especially dedicated to learning about FODMAPs and sharing your knowledge with others.

Sarah Prusinowski was the editor of this book, with additional proofreading services provided by Jennifer Caven. As a self-published author, my hands are the last ones to work on the manuscript, and I take full responsibility for any errors that may have crept into the text after they so ably did their jobs. This is my fourth self-published book, and I would like to thank the technical support team at Create Space and KDP for their ready assistance. Unsung heroes of our day include contributors to the Create Space Community, the KDP Support Forum, the Open Office.org Community Forum, and various bloggers for the time they devote to helping others solve technical problems and learn to negotiate the self-publishing process.

This book is dedicated to my husband, Paul Catsos, who has eaten every meal I've put in front of him for over 30 years. (The one exception was an ill-advised plate of fried smelts, little fish you cook and eat whole—it's a Maine thing.) Paul, thank you for sharing my table and my life since the day we met in the kitchen at Cornell Dining. Here's to thirty more years. Cheers!

ABOUT THE AUTHOR

Patsy Danehy Catsos, M.S., R.D.N, L.D., is a nutritionist on a mission to reduce pain and improve quality of life for people with digestive health issues, especially irritable bowel syndrome (IBS) and small intestinal bacterial overgrowth (SIBO). The days of over-generalized advice for people with stomach problems are over. Advising everyone with IBS to "eat more fiber" and "avoid red meat, alcohol, and caffeine" just doesn't cut it anymore. Patsy doesn't believe in one-size-fits-all diets; she helps you discover the diet that works for you.

Her trailblazing book, *IBS—Free at Last!* (Pond Cove Press, 2009) introduced U.S. health care providers and consumers to an exciting and effective dietary program for finding and eliminating food triggers for irritable bowel syndrome. In 2013, the second edition of her book was translated into Spanish. Patsy is the editor of the blog IBSfree.net, and an expert contributor to Sharecare.com, an interactive social Q/A platform created by Jeff Arnold and Dr. Mehmet Oz, in partnership with Harpo Studios, HSW International, Sony Pictures Television, and Discovery Communications. She has been consulted for expert comments in numerous web and print publications, including *WebMD*, *Today's Dietitian*, *SpryLiving.com*, *Bloomberg.com*, *Blisstree.com*, *EmpowHer.com*, *CatchingHealth.com*, *Clinical Nutrition Insight* and *Consumer Reports Shop Smart Magazine*. Patsy provides continuing professional education to other dietitians on the delivery of the FODMAP elimination diet.

Ms. Catsos earned a B.S. in Nutritional Science from Cornell University and an M.S. in Nutrition at Boston University. She completed her internship at Boston's Beth Israel Hospital. Ms. Catsos maintains a private practice in Portland, Maine. She is a professional member of the Crohn's and Colitis Foundation of American and the Academy of Nutrition and Dietetics, and she is a past-president of the Maine Academy of Nutrition and Dietetics.

Patsy looks forward to corresponding with readers through her blog, www.ibsfree.net. Use the "comments" link available at the bottom of each blog post to ask questions, let her know how this book has helped you, or share information that might help others. Follow @CatsosIBSFreeRD on Twitter, pcatsos on Pinterest and "like" IBSFree on Facebook to be notified about new blog posts, FODMAP-friendly foods, and other items of interest.

INDEX

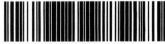

5774507R00072

Printed in Great Britain
by Amazon.co.uk, Ltd.,
Marston Gate.